Midwifery in China (中国助产)

The first book to present the history, ideas, life and works of Chinese midwives and birth attendants, this volume seeks to encapsulate and explain the changing ideas about the practice of midwifery in China.

Using participant observations and interviews, it examines each phase of the development of midwifery in depth. Providing a systematic study of the existing literature and contemporary national health policies, it analyses the factors contributing to the current demise of midwifery in China, such as the absence of national regulation, high standards of education and national midwives' associations. Furthermore, it argues that China's national statistics in the past six decades demonstrate clear evidence that minimising maternal mortality rates will only happen through wider availability of services, rather than through obstetric technology or facility-based care. Ultimately, therefore, this book supports the view that humanity and midwifery will survive to overcome domination by both technology and market forces and that economic growth and medical technology alone will not be sufficient in providing effective healthcare.

This book is an indispensable resource for the study of Chinese midwifery, both in theory and in practice. As such it will be useful to students and scholars of midwifery, women's health, sociology and culture and society in China.

Ngai Fen Cheung (张毅芬) is an independent midwifery researcher. She is also the honorary permanent expert at the Shijiazhuang Obstetric and Gynaecology Hospital, China, and adviser to the Chinese Midwifery Expert Committee, Chinese Maternal and Child Health Association.

Rosemary Mander (曼德昳) is Emeritus Professor of Midwifery at the University of Edinburgh, UK. She has practised as a midwife in the UK, both independently and in the National Health Service.

Routledge Contemporary China Series

For more information about this series, please visit: www.routledge.com/
Routledge-Contemporary-China-Series/book-series/SE0768

Midwifery in China (中国助产)

**Ngai Fen Cheung (张毅芬) and
Rosemary Mander (曼德跞)**

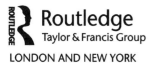

Routledge
Taylor & Francis Group

LONDON AND NEW YORK

First published 2018 by Routledge

2 Park Square, Milton Park, Abingdon, Oxfordshire OX14 4RN
52 Vanderbilt Avenue, New York, NY 10017

Routledge is an imprint of the Taylor & Francis Group, an informa business

First issued in paperback 2020

British Library Cataloguing-in-Publication Data
A catalogue record for this book is available from the British Library

Library of Congress Cataloging-in-Publication Data
Names: Cheung, Ngai Fen, author. | Mander, Rosemary, author.
Title: Midwifery in China / Ngai Fen Cheung and Rosemary Mander.
Description: Milton Park, Abingdon ; New York, NY : Routledge, 2018. |
    Includes bibliographical references and index.
Identifiers: LCCN 2018002762 | ISBN 9780815357414 (hardback) |
    ISBN 9781351124522 (ebook)
Subjects: LCSH: Midwifery—China—History. | Midwives—China—
    History.
Classification: LCC RG950 .C48 2018 | DDC 618.200951—dc23
LC record available at https://lccn.loc.gov/2018002762

ISBN: 978-0-8153-5741-4 (hbk)
ISBN: 978-0-367-58940-0 (pbk)

Typeset in Times New Roman
by Apex CoVantage, LLC

Contents

Figures

Tables

Acknowledgements

This book has been more than a decade in the making. We, the authors, would like to express our gratitude to those who have helped in the preparation of this book. This applies particularly to the generous cooperation of Chinese midwives and birth attendants who were interviewed over the years for this project.

We are extremely grateful for the sponsorship received from the British Academy; the University of Edinburgh; the Royal Society of Edinburgh; the Carnegie Trust; *Hángzhōu* Qianjian Specially Appointed Expert; the International Confederation of Midwives; Shijiazhuang Maternal and Children's Hospital; the Pioneering Development Fund for the Returned Chinese Overseas Scholar from *Hángzhōu* Human Resources, China; Social Security Bureau of *Hángzhōu*, China; the Nursing School of *Hángzhōu* Normal University, China; and *Hángzhōu* First People's Hospital, *Zhèjiāng*, China.

The authors' gratitude also goes to Professor Jen-der Lee, Professor Angela Ki Che Leung, Professor Charlotte Furth, Professor Lesley Barclay, Professor Denis Walsh, Professor Nicky Leap, Dr Lindsay Reid, Dr Alison Nuttall, Dr Iain Hutchison the anonymous reviewers and the late and much-lamented Sheila Kitzinger.

We would like to express our gratitude to Professor Fu Wei, Ms Wang Xiaoli, Dr Gao Yan, Dr Zhu Chunzhi, Dr Wang Zhihua, Dr Li Hejiang, Ms Guo Honghua, Ms Geng Linghua, Ms Cai Dincui, Ms Long Suqiong, Ms Ma Dongmei, and Ms Wang Yan.

Above all, NFC owes a special debt to her husband, Dr Anshi Pan, who provided her with understanding, academic discussions and unending generosity of support, without which she would never have been able to carry out and complete this work. Her thanks also go to her daughter, Rebecca, who provided the first-hand experience on childbearing, childbirth and childrearing for her as a mother, midwife and midwifery researcher and who had to learn to live with a forever preoccupied mother.

1 Introduction

China has made tremendous achievements in many fields since it committed to reform in the 1980s. There have been new developments in medical care and technology. From 1978 to 2010, the number of hospitals and primary health care institutions increased more than thirteen-fold to 922,627, while the population increased by only about 40% or 1,337 million (Countrymeters 2015). The number of physicians increased from 1.07 per 1,000 population to 1.79, and nurses, from 0.4 to 1.52. In maternity, infant mortality dropped from 31.6 to 13.1 per 1,000. Maternal mortality fell from 100 to 30 per 100,000 (Koblinsky et al. 2000; National Bureau of Statistics of China 2003: 7; CMoH 2011b; China News Network 2011).

These statistics refute some traditional sayings, such as

> in childbirth ten women would die, only one would survive

and

> childbirth was only one foot on earth, the other in hell or in the coffin.
> (Lee 2008: 13; Yan 1989)

These achievements are associated with social stability, rapid economic development, improvement of living standards and advances in and increased popularity of medical technology.

Rethinking development: one example

As medical expertise has developed rapidly in China, phenomena have emerged which need attention and more thought. Among these is the overuse of medical technology in childbirth. The caesarean operation is a very appropriate example of such overuse.

In 1960s Shanghai the caesarean rate was 4.7%, and it increased to 44% in 1998. In many hospitals in other cities caesarean rates reached 40% in the 1990s, with some reaching over 60% (Cai et al. 1998; Huang 2000; Dai 2004). Between 2007 and 2008, World Health Organization (WHO) conducted a randomised survey in nine Asian countries. The study showed that during this period China's caesarean rate was 46.2%, of which 9.3% and 2.4%, respectively, were found without either antenatal or intrapartum medical indications. These rates were the highest among the nine countries, whose average caesarean rate was 27.3%. The lowest was 14.7% in Cambodia. The average Asian caesarean rate without antenatal or intrapartum indication was 1.4% and 1.5%, with the lowest of 0.1% and 0% in Japan (WHO 2010). Apart from the overuse of caesarean in China, there were also indications of the excessive or unnecessary use of medical interventions in childbirth, such as unnecessary routine pubic shaving, enema, rupture of membranes and excessive use of oxytocin and pharmacological analgesia.

The widespread application of medical technology in maternity care has demonstrated the richness of health care resources. But the excessive use of technology means overemphasis on efficiency, which may be iatrogenic (causing harm to women and babies in the course of treatment). It is, simultaneously, a waste of resources. Medical science and technology were invented to treat disease from day one. Childbirth is a physiological phenomenon. There should not be any routine reliance on medicine during childbirth. If, at a time when living conditions, physical health and living standards have improved generally, half or even just 27% (Lumbiganon et al. 2010) of the women still have to rely on medical technology during birth, it cannot be denied that there is something wrong. Much has been written recently to warn of the dangers of caesarean to women and babies (Mander 2007). A Swedish study showed that maternal mortality associated with caesarean was more than 12 times higher than with vaginal birth. Although this may include maternal disease-related factors, it provides a perspective indicating the dangers associated with caesarean. Appropriate use of caesarean is life-saving in complicated childbirth. Its use without medical indications does not reduce, but instead increases, maternal mortality (Huang 2000).The WHO found that a caesarean rate of not more than 10% could be justified by research evidence (Beech 2008). Variations related to global differences in living and health conditions.

China's capacity to reduce maternal and infant mortality after the 1950s, including developments in other aspects of health care especially in the rural areas, was highly praised by the international community (CMoH et al. 2006: 14). An international study has suggested that strong political leadership and a commitment to equal access to health services for all facilitated China's achievement (Koblinsky et al. 2000: 41). The Chinese policy of focusing health resources on rural areas during this period was successful, even though an in-depth evaluation of many issues is still needed.

International background

In its process of industrialisation and modernisation China is not unique in overusing medical technology to control childbirth. In America's modernisation in the late 19th century, midwives were systematically replaced by obstetricians. Fear was engendered among 'the delicate upper middle class women' to make them scared of childbirth, labour pain and associated risks and that 'American society has had a profound fear of nature, and a strong desire for medical technology with an uneasy trust of it' (Davis-Floyd & Sargent 1997: 9, 11; Davis-Floyd 1992, 1994). The idea of medical control of childbirth in the US was so overwhelming that up until the 1950s, 'twilight sleep' (a form of general anaesthesia) was used for women experiencing vaginal birth. Forceps and episiotomy were routinely used (Donnison 1988: 201; Arms 1994: 1). In Britain, the Edinburgh obstetrician Sir James Young Simpson (1811–1870) was the first to use chloroform in 1847. He claimed to use it to free women from their labour pain. In 1948, the UK National Health Service was established, followed by the government encouraging women to give birth only in hospitals. The medical lobby persuaded the government of the greater safety for women and babies in obstetric consultant maternity units. In hospitals, as medical science and obstetric technology were developed, the tendency increased for obstetric professionals to use them.

In the West, maternity care in history has been overshadowed by the gender struggle. During the 18th and 19th centuries' industrialisation and development of science and technology, Western European women were perceived as congenitally lacking the intellectual capacity possessed by men in reasoning and decision-making, preventing their entry into, for example, medicine. Even midwifery, traditionally a women's occupation, was taken over by men as medical practice became more specialised and new devices, for example, obstetric forceps, were invented. Men were thought to be the right people to use these techniques. Male midwives became fashionable (Donnison 1988: 34–52, 80). To the patriarchal medical establishment, women's reproductive power was a disability, being the root of female inferiority (Oakley 1980: 12). Others thought that it was an 'inefficient womb', especially in the first birth, that justified the use of medical technology (Donnison 1988: 193). The discrimination against and prejudice towards women and their bodily functioning had reached a pitiful extent.

Since the 1960s, development of feminist movements and more in-depth research in sociology and anthropology into medicine and reproduction, woman's adverse experiences in childbirth and in gender politics have attracted much attention. Scholars of social and cultural anthropology who conducted research in the traditional societies in developing countries had found that, although these societies lacked the so-called high tech interventions, they nevertheless had their own effective forms of midwifery care in childbirth and labour. Examples include external cephalic conversion, walking to ease the discomfort of uterine contractions and shorten labour, standing or kneeling to take advantage of gravity, changing position to help labouring women feel better and cauterisation of the umbilical cord stump. More important, women in traditional societies gave birth in their own familiar environment. It was less hindrance to communication during labour (e.g., no language barrier), and midwives were more caring. Women were under no hospital 'routine' restriction. Since they could move about and change positions as they felt like it, labour progressed more smoothly. From a Western medical point of view, these methods of facilitating birth were often seen as 'backward' or 'unscientific' (Jordan 1987).

By contrast, the over-provision of medical technology in developed industrialised countries threatened the well-being of the mother and baby. It disregarded the individual character of women in childbirth and of their specific sociocultural background and environment. It cannot be said that these practices are 'scientific' and 'advanced'. Anthropologists also pointed out that childbirth has almost never been a simple biophysical behaviour. Childbirth is socially and culturally shaped universally (Jordan 1993: 1; Davis-Floyd & Sargent 1997: 1). This view has profound implications in so-called science and the theory and practice of maternity and midwifery.

Understanding medicine and midwifery

The unnecessary overuse of medical technology and the medical control of childbirth and labour have been labelled the 'medicalisation' of childbirth (Lock & Nguyen 2010: 48, 68), or the 'medical model' of maternity care (Rothman 1982: 34; Downe 2008: 191) in the sociology of medicine and health. Some scholars even called these the 'technocratic model' (Davis-Floyd et al. 2009: 456–60). The main features of this model are pregnancy and labour as potentially pathological crises in women's lives and losses in body function; the body as a machine, separated from the mind; hospitals as factories; babies as products; childbirth to a strict schedule; labour pain as an unacceptable problem; women as needing to be acted on, not as the actor; only the obstetrician's knowledge is correct, and he leads the birth; hospital is hierarchical; services are economically effective (Davis-Floyd et al. 2009: 16, 442, 456–60).

The 'technocrats' in maternity care developed on the basis of medical science and technology exported from industrially advanced societies. The export often brought an imbalance of technological capacity and power between the exporting and the importing societies so that such technology is often seen as advanced. They would become symbols of 'progress' and 'advance', whether they have use-value in local conditions or not (see Jordan 1987). On a deeper level, such so-called advanced and sophisticated technology carried with it social and cultural values, and even factors of biophysiological differences. For example, Inuit women in North America usually have quick births because of their diet, lifestyle and environment, so a care plan following the science based on West European biophysiological characteristics is unsuitable for Inuit women (Lock & Nguyen 2010: 48). Physiological labour pain has carried even more social and cultural values, making the pain of uterine contractions felt and accepted differently by women in different societies and cultures.

The problem of the medical model as applied to childbirth has illustrated the complexity of childbirth. Childbirth is a healthy, normal, physiological process, but it is also a varied and changing process. With scientific 'positivism' as its starting point, medical technology seeks certainty in the normal uncertainty of childbirth; for example, only generalised research data are used to determine what is normal and what is pathological. This approach denies precisely the individual character and the uncertainty of childbirth (Downe 2008: 1–27). From a medical point of view, uncertainty is a problem and, therefore, to obstetricians normality is an outcome, not a process; only after the child is born can the labour be considered 'normal'. This way of looking at things leads to the use of medical technology and very often defensively; for medical staff, technology removes uncertainty, brings clarity and becomes crucial should disputes arise.

Childbirth is so important for human society that it should be emphasised that women in pregnancy are attended to, cared for and assisted by other women. This is an indispensable civilising aspect of human society, even though such civilised acts are practised differently with different spiritual orientations across different societies and cultures as they develop. Midwifery is a very old occupation, certainly older than recorded history (Donnison 1988: 11) or as old as society itself. The development of medical science and technology has not only led to too much unnecessary intervention but also resulted in a takeover of midwifery as a female profession by medical technology as dominated by men under patriarchal ideologies. Some scholars have even suggested that male-dominated medicine's hostility to women is based on fear of female reproductive power. The fear results in a desire to control normal childbirth by such medical technology and to exclude female-dominated midwifery, just as happened in North American industrial societies up to the late 20th century (Ehrenreich & English 1973; Ehrenreich 1976).

Other studies point out that medical technology has not completely played the key role in the changes in health status, in the elimination of some diseases, and in the decline of mortality rates. A notorious example is tuberculosis, whose decline pre-dated the discovery of Bacillus Calmette-Guerin (BCG). There is a close link to rising living standards, including better food, nutrition, water and housing (Scambler 2008: 6). The fall in maternal and infant mortality is comparable. The contrast between the achievements made in maternity care in China before and after 1980 also explains it. The flaws of medical technology in maternity care, and the social reality that it needs to face, have highlighted the importance of midwifery which is mainly practised by women. It is wrong to simply regard the practices of traditional midwives and home birth as backward, and assume that childbirth must be supervised by medical technology. It is even more erroneous to look at midwifery from the point of view of medical patriarchy. The practices in some European countries, such as the Netherlands, in their industrial era have also pointed to a lesser position for medical technology in maternity care.

Similarly, in Nordic countries, such as Sweden, where maternal and infant mortality rates are among the lowest in the world (2008: 4.6/100,000), midwives have provided care for almost all births (De Vries et al. 2009). Since the end of 20th century, the important role of midwives in childbirth has been more and more recognised. It was in America, where medical technology was the most popular, that scholars had first pointed out the need for a 'midwifery model' in childbirth (Davis-Floyd et al. 2009: 442). 'The State of the World's Midwifery 2014' (UNFPA et al. 2014) developed from the first call to action; the 2011 report shows that only 4 of 73 low- and middle-income countries have a midwifery workforce that is able to meet the universal need for the essential intervention for sexual, reproductive, maternal and newborn health. It proposed to strengthen the training for skilled birth attendants and midwives in countries where maternal and infant mortality is still very high (such as Afghanistan, where the maternal mortality rate in 2008 was 1,575/100,000). To enhance the public services of midwifery is a strategic initiative for worldwide maternal and infant health (UNFPA et al. 2011, 2014).

Objectives and significance of this book

Since the 1980s maternal and infant mortality in China has not declined as quickly as the development of medical technology has increased. Infant mortality remains unchanged, but some Asian countries with similar or slower economic development, such as Malaysia, Thailand, Vietnam and Sri Lanka, have achieved faster progress. By 2005, the mortality of children under five years in China was even higher than in these countries. Of maternal deaths, 75% were avoidable, which further confirms the inappropriate, unreasonable and imbalanced use of obstetric technology (CMoH et al. 2006: 14, 24).

China is a populous country with immense regional differences in many aspects. This is a reality, and this reality can become more salient amid the new economic developments. To some extent, this reality may explain the inappropriate, unreasonable and imbalanced provision of maternity care and obstetric technology which affected China's progress in overall statistical terms since the 1980s. However, in a firm and integrated political and sociocultural entity such as China, there should not have been an intrinsic relationship between this reality and maternity care. Furthermore, the Chinese civilisation is an advanced society and culture of long historical standing, which includes, among other things, the well-known holistic Chinese medicine and the philosophy of health. If childbirth has never been a pure biological and physiological process, this civilisation is bound to have held a key to childbirth and its care. The holistic philosophy of medicine and health care has the logic of bringing humanity, culture and society, biophysiology, natural environment and health into one whole. As biophysiological, medical sciences develop, the holistic idea should have greater evolutionary potential. Under this potential lies the answer to the question of the development of Chinese maternity care. It has been shown that the medical model of care provided no answer, but brought instead problems; therefore, on the basis of the Chinese civilisation of culture and society, to further and greatly develop midwifery as a way forward. It has been clearly shown (Renfrew et al. 2014) that a vital mechanism in leading to increasing well-being and reducing adverse events is midwives' involvement. They can change the whole philosophy of how birth is looked at and cared for.

This understanding formed a base for us in research and practice to develop a midwife-led unit called 'Homely Birth Unit' from 2007 to 2009. The practice of the unit confirms the role that midwives can play in the management and enhancement of normality in childbirth and labour (Cheung et al. 2011a, b). This service model has brought higher levels of satisfaction to women and their families, midwives and medical staff alike. With the ideas, research and practice, we ask further questions. China is an ancient, civilised country, and there is no doubt that midwifery is an important part of this civilisation. What then is midwifery's history, evolutionary path and current state of affairs? How did childbirth happen and how has it been facilitated? Who were these carers? What do Chinese women want? At the same time, under the new historical and social circumstances, what new understandings of this history and evolution should we reach? With new understandings of history, how do we rebuild and improve midwifery? These are exactly the questions to which we are seeking answers. This cyclical thinking from history to the present and from the present to history is a very basic way of investigation. It can be said to be a tool to improve social institutions and their management continuously. In dealing with the issue of midwifery, we are using this tool. So between 2004 and 2013 when the 'Homely Birth Unit' was developing and improving, we began investigating the history and current state of Chinese midwifery in some cities and villages in central and south-west China. The main part of this book is built on this study.

What is the significance of asking these questions about midwifery? This is, of course, closely linked to the above discussion of the importance of midwifery. The central purpose of this book is to uncover and clarify from its historical development that midwifery is a key profession in enhancing normal childbirth and in safeguarding maternal and infant health. To develop the midwifery profession, an understanding of the issues concerning the history and the current state of affairs of midwifery is an important starting point. We are also going to indicate that research into enhancing normal childbirth by midwives should be developed. The professional midwifery service can only be established and developed, substantiated and upgraded as a highly educated discipline on such a basis. The significance of this book also lies in its initiative to explore the professional history of midwifery and therefore demonstrates a further understanding of midwifery practice.

An enlightened review of the development of midwifery will only serve as an inspiration to develop more research into the care needed to enhance normal childbirth, into midwifery as a professional service and into its professional training and education. Our review and survey of midwifery's past practice are closely related to the professional identity of and fulfilment for midwives, which are important factors in developing and consolidating this service.

Midwifery practice encountered gender-political issues in its relation to the progress and advancement of medical science. There are other more complicated issues of social relations, sociocultural values in maternity and its care to consider. This means that the ideology and ways of thinking in childbirth care cannot be overlooked. These ideologies and ways of thinking directly related to a view of women's reproductive power, the status of their health and well-being, the sociocultural values of childbirth and values of midwifery itself. The review and rethinking of midwifery practice and its current state therefore involves the ideological debate on childbirth and its care. It can be argued that such a debate is inevitable for maternity services and midwifery to develop and to modernise.

Structure and design

The book is divided into three parts to discuss the issues raised on midwifery practice in China: (1) history and development, (2) current state and issues and (3) prospects for midwives and midwifery.

Part I, 'A history of Chinese midwifery and its development', introduces chronologically the history and development of Chinese midwifery in four chapters and gives readers an overview of the history and development of maternity in China. It provides a framework of understanding in terms of time and historical data. At the same time we discuss historical issues and their impact on midwifery development from our current viewpoints. The last chapter introduces and discusses the development, research and practice of the midwife-led 'Homely Birth Unit'. This new practice is judged in equal historical terms. This part serves as a critique of history and tradition. It will be significant in renewing thinking about the history of midwifery practice.

Part II, 'The present state and issues in Chinese midwifery', in three chapters, examines three issues: 'professionalisation', 'modernisation' and 'marginalisation'. We think that for midwifery to become an important part of health care, these issues are what we need to understand. These are concepts which cause concern and are discussed in other industrial societies in different social and cultural contexts. In the midwifery service with China's particular social and cultural background, the presence of and social aspirations in these issues have their own characteristics. However, as today the world communities become more integrated, different social and cultural values, ideologies, theories and practices of science and technology infiltrate more into economic, social and cultural life, the current state and development of midwifery are no longer isolated phenomena; perhaps they have never been isolated phenomena. We need to see development from the perspective of social and cultural exchange and impact and reveal differences and similarities of midwifery practices of different social and cultural backgrounds. The current state of midwifery and related issues cannot be separated from historical development; therefore, the understanding of history and tradition is integrated throughout the three parts of the book.

What more rational shape of the maternity care and midwifery service with modern goals can develop in China, how the complexity theory and the issues of the so-called 'marginalisation' can be overcome in the division of work and professional co-operation will be discussed in depth in this part.

In Part III, 'The prospects for midwives and midwifery in China', relying on the interviews, historical data and literature, we recount the personal experience, the professional sense and understanding of past and contemporary individual midwives. Through these experiences and ideas, we aim to reveal more issues facing midwifery as an important service in health care. By relating this part with the issues touched on in the last two parts, especially Part II, we put forward our view concerning the prospects for the development of midwifery in China.

Part I

History and development

This book is divided into three parts. The first part addresses the history of Chinese midwifery, introducing chronologically the development of Chinese midwifery in four chapters. An overall picture is presented of the growth of maternity care in China. The fourth chapter introduces and discusses the introduction of the midwife-led 'Homely Birth Unit' and judges it in historical terms. This critique of history and tradition will be significant in renewing ideas about the history of midwifery practice.

We may say that midwifery is as old as human society, as has been suggested by the British midwifery historian Donnison (1988: 11). To understand Chinese midwifery, a good start is to learn about its history. Four chapters are devoted in this section to present the ideas and the development of Chinese midwifery before and after integration with European midwifery practice at the beginning of the 20th century. The organisation of the material has both chronological and thematic elements. We have tried to emphasise, on one hand, the continuity and transformation of ideas and practices in Chinese midwifery and, on the other, the impact of the changes in the past and the present practices. Where relevant we stress disjunction too, when medical and health professional authorities had rejected midwifery practices and then changed their minds again.

History will be indispensable to constructing a theory of Chinese midwifery. Some disciplinary historians have suggested perspectives to look at the history of a discipline either as a sequence of events, a succession of time frames, a system of ideas, a set of parallel regional traditions or a process of constant change (Barnard 2000: 12). These may serve as good suggestions for us to start. We look at the history of Chinese midwifery in a succession of time frames, which is, in fact, the chronological method mentioned earlier. We also see Chinese midwifery as a regional tradition, which was in a process of constant change. This means we are also making comparisons, comparing it with other traditions, such as the European ones, and with its own past. Our thematic method to discuss the development of and change in Chinese midwifery in Part II is just such a perspective. Did Chinese midwifery have a system of ideas? The answer is both yes and no. We say yes because as a regional tradition, Chinese midwifery must have had its ideological content. We say no because in Chinese academic history, midwifery had not held a disciplinary position, and therefore, this content did not constitute a disciplinary system of ideas. In their practices to look after birthing women throughout the ages, midwives, being traditional (*chǎnpó*) or modern (*zhùchǎnshì*), must have accumulated rich midwifery experiences from which ideas could be established. Although midwifery was dealing with a very important aspect of life, childbirth, it was very often the other learning in history, such as medicine and philosophy, that had provided or prescribed ideas to its practices. There is a historical reason for the discipline of midwifery to develop in multidisciplinary terms. In comparison to medicine, midwifery was much less documented in Chinese history. In a sense, while we are inquiring into Chinese midwifery, whether as an academic discipline or as a professional practice, we are also reconstructing it as such. The discussions in Part I are part of such a historical contribution.

2 Research considerations

The theme of this book is the perception and position of maternity care and care providers in both ancient and modern China in relation to current maternity services. History and modernity are used as tools to facilitate this assessment.

History not only means things that happened in the past but also means the study of or learning about those things (Jordanova 2006: 13). It is a part of our triple construction of reality in time: the past, the present and the future. In such a construction, we, the authors, have necessarily rendered a transforming power to our concept of history. It is by such a power that we are able to change or to transform ourselves and our societies. If history is what we did in the past, modernity is what we are doing in the present. But what we are doing in the present is no less problematic than what we did in the past. We often think of drawing lessons from the past, but we are just as much being inspired by the past. Obviously, we are looking for hindsight to enhance our understanding and retrospection. If we feel that hindsight is found appropriately, this finding lies in the way that we have learned and understood our history. We can say that such a way is the progress of history, and it is modernity. In our view, then, modernity is not about beliefs in the superiority of rational thought over emotion, in the ability of technology and science to solve human problems and so on, as have been suggested (Haralambos & Holborn 2008: 7). Modernity is about continuous understanding of ourselves, our relations with each other and with our time and space, others' time and spaces and the progress of history itself.

'History' and 'modernity' are then two paradoxical concepts; each is as much relying on the other as it is against the other. Using this paradox, we are uncovering and discussing the meanings in the development of Chinese midwifery.

To achieve these objectives, the present study was conducted in six stages, by which we approached the question of how childbirth has been facilitated by Chinese midwifery: (1) literature review, (2) ethical approval, (3) participant observation, (4) semi-structured and unstructured interviews, (5) a regional comparison and (6) the data collected were analysed in the light of the filter of 'sceptical subjectivity' (Haralambos & Holborn 2008: 681), using a mixture of sociological and anthropological approaches.

Literature review

The materials are arranged chronologically and thematically.

Historical literature overview

The Chinese have a recorded history of about 3,000 years. An imperial 'Four Libraries' were built in the 18th century, aimed at collecting all the literature. A library system with 'four divisions' (*sì-bù*; see Guide to Chinese Words and Pronunciation – hereafter, Guide – The *Pīnyīn* system) and the tones were first established by the imperial scholars between the 3rd and 4th centuries (see Guide – Chinese glossary for all Chinese appellations used in this book and their meanings). The 'four divisions' became 'four libraries' (*sì-kù*) in the 7th century. An encyclopaedia of 'Comprehensive Chinese Classics' was compiled in the early 15th century. By the 18th century, on the basis of these developments, the imperial collection, some of which was taken from private hands, reached 79,218 volumes including 3,471 subjects. The emperor then had those valuable and orthodox ones copied and organised into the so-called Four Imperial Libraries with All Books (*sì-kù-quán-shū*; Yang 1967).

In the development of *sì-kù-quán-shū*, we may notice that these materials had been laboriously copied again and again from the original manuscripts at a time when they were still available. We also find what we are actually dealing with are copies of copies and copies of originals. Over the years, in the process of repeated copying, various 'accidents' may have altered the original texts. Although it is not the purpose for us to discuss these accidents here, some typical instances are indicated in the discussion.

First, understanding the original is crucial to the process of accurate copying. These books were copied many times for different purposes and in different Chinese dynasties. The meanings and many expressions have been changed with the development of the society and its language. It is not only punctuation but also some words that are likely to have been lost or corrupted in the process of socio-political changes; whole lines or groups of lines can be lost, for example, the development of punctuation in Chinese and the omission of minor words. A similar phenomenon can be seen today in hastily prepared printed works, such as daily newspapers.

Second, language corruption may occur through a scribe's good intentions to improve on the original. For example, this takes the form of modernising its writing style and updating a text which sounded archaic. The temptation to do this must have been strong. Such modernisation is disappointing to those of us who hope to find interesting early forms of words. Most dangerous is the scribe who knows, or thinks he or she knows, more than the original author and who succumbs to the temptation to exhibit his or her knowledge.

One final general consideration is the manuscripts' age. Much attention is always and rightly paid to the actual date of the manuscripts with which we are working. People, in general, might well imagine that, faced with a number of copies of the same text, of varying date, the historian always prefers the earliest, but this is not necessarily so. What matters is not the date of the manuscript but the source behind it. This is true even when dealing with variant manuscripts of the same ancient original. The first task here is to discover the nature of the sources which lie behind them.

However, within such a seemingly mammoth literary culture, childbirth, birthing practices, women's history and what we now know as midwifery consist of very few lines or pages, usually subsumed under traditional Chinese medicine dealing with women's diseases. Recent Chinese medical and social historians (Fu et al. 1982; Liang 1983; Leung 2000; Lee 2008) have made attempts to reinterpret Chinese historical materials. In reviewing these materials, one must, first of all, ask, 'Was there any "midwifery" in Chinese history?'

Although midwifery was not a significant subject in Chinese history, the appellation given to the maternity carers may yet give us clues as to the existence of midwifery and the social status of midwives in Chinese history. In Chinese historical materials, there are clear indications that childbirth was, first, very important but dangerous; second, that women's health was important to ensure that birth took place without danger; third, that 'medicine-men' or 医者 (Lee 2008:127, 358) had technical authority over the birth; and, fourth, that other birth attendants were often nobodies (e.g., a childbirth story quoted in Lee [2003]). But, as Lee has shown, when female attendants were dismissed by medicine-men was exactly when a midwife's techniques would have enhanced the birth.

In reviewing Chinese historical materials, we know that these materials were largely produced by an elite. Therefore, the exclusive medicine-man's supervision of childbirth described in literature did not necessarily mean such supervision was available to all Chinese women. In Chinese birthing culture, men were forbidden entry into the birthing room. Medical supervision, if there was any, was always conducted by men away from the birthing room. The absence of medicine-men meant that birth attendants or traditional midwives would be at childbirth.

Traditional Chinese medicine believes in the natural balance of *yīn-yáng* (see Chapter 3; *Wáng* 762; Unschuld 1985). Women giving birth were seen as following the natural order. Human birth was compared to cattle going through the same process (Lee 2008: 3–4). A birth complication was thought to be due to the presence of too many attendants. While no Chinese books on midwifery have ever been written, Chinese traditional medical books on pregnancy and birth focus on pathology. To reconstruct a history of Chinese midwifery, we need to explore other related literature, including those about birthing culture, women's life stories, diet (as Chinese diet often relates to health care) and even fortune telling (childbirth was always too important to ignore a divination).

In this study, we choose to identify and use historical evidence, in three facets: what actually happened, speculation and interpretation. Historians generally recognise that history is largely written (Carr 1986: 15). We may never know what exactly happened in history. With careful consideration of a historical source in different aspects, such as the author, the literary tradition in question and the historical period in which the event took place, however, we may approach historical events as closely as possible. Speculative evidence is based on our contemporary knowledge structure. A social theory such as a structuralist or functionalist paradigm can enhance our capacity to speculate about a historical event. Interpretation is done through the perspectives of the scholars who did the interpretation. These three facets of evidence are interconnected. So with a particular piece of evidence, we may identify what actually happened in some aspects but speculate and interpret the event in other aspects.

Chinese midwifery and its development

In the second part of the literature review, we identify the key historical stages in the development of midwifery in Chinese history. Recent Chinese medical historians (mainly Taiwanese) have provided some useful material and insights into such developments (Fu et al. 1982; Liang 1983; Leung 2000; Lee 2003, 2005, 2008). We reinterpret these materials and discuss them from sociological perspectives, such as the social status of midwives in Chinese history, the legitimacy of the practice of midwifery in historical China and so on. There is scope here for further investigation in social history, but this would involve in-depth assessment of medieval and pre-modern Chinese societies (see Timeline) and geographical boundaries. The reinterpretation of the historical development of Chinese midwifery provides sufficient clues to answer the question we asked at the beginning of this chapter.

Issues arising – sociological influences

The third part of the literature review in this study is to identify sociological concerns which may answer the question, 'Do the Chinese need midwifery?' Since the end of the 20th century, in one way or another, China has followed the industrial path that has been taken by Western European countries, even though it is striving to build an economic and social order in its own way. We can nevertheless anticipate that, apart from its traditional cultures, the Chinese will face social problems similar to those experienced in European societies. Chinese social historians have been largely re-interpreting Chinese historical data on medicine and birth, whereas social scientists of a European sociological and anthropological tradition have been trying to pin down a Chinese conception of pregnancy and childbirth, through a cultural approach (Furth 1987). Yet we have found a rigour in Euro-American sociological traditions that would enable us to approach societies as complex as Chinese society through different aspects of its social life. Therefore, Chinese midwifery practices will not only be seen as a problem to meet the demand for a birth or to meet obstetric technologies but will also be seen as related to other sociological issues. These issues are balance of power, interest in different social strata, the meaning of modernity, institutional contradictions, customary behaviour, the relationships between health workers, gender, tradition and the public's ambivalent feelings toward Chinese midwives.

We adopt a historical and sociological approach in this chapter in that we see a historical approach which can have social consequences. While history may imply changes, these changes will often affect a particular social identity. The varied fortunes of Chinese midwifery are a case in point. Chinese midwives may be seen, and see themselves, in a better social position through this sociological perspective.

The research

A number of approaches were used to collect the data and they are discussed here. Of course, ethical approval was obtained from the institutions where the researchers work and permission to access the hospitals and midwives was granted by management. Ethical conventions were conscientiously followed throughout.

Participant observation

Participant observation is used in the study (Jordanova 2006: 44–7) to enable us to be a part of the culture and be sensitive to the problems of meaning and context through the process of interpreting and sharing the experience of the respondents. Also known as ethnography, fieldwork or field research (Junker 1960; Burgess 1982; Parahoo 2006), it covers varieties of participation, observation, informal interviewing and any other methods that are available to the researcher to tackle a research problem. A participant observer adopts a multitude of social roles, trying to understand people under investigation objectively from their own frame of reference and/or to understand them subjectively through the observer's own involvement with the culture. It is through this process of interpretation of the experienced culture that the observer discovers meanings in the data (Bruyn 1966: 27–8). In a narrow sense, according to Seymour-Smith (1986: 216), participant observation now may be only one of a set of research techniques, not including interviews.

Critics of participant observation point out its possible biases, such as the lack of adequate criteria of proof and its tendency to produce purely descriptive accounts. Various writers suggest ways to overcome the limitations of this approach. Malinowski advocated extensive periods of fieldwork to minimise the effects of the fieldworker's presence and to permit a full appreciation of cultural meanings and the social structure of the group with all its functional interrelation between customs and beliefs (cited in Seymour-Smith 1986: 216). Many writers suggest the use of diverse methods to approach a research problem and to assess the validity of the research, for example, Stacey's (1969) 'combined operations', Denzin's (1970) 'triangulation' and Burgess's (1982) 'multiple strategies'. These methods have one thing in common – that the application of multiple sets of data, strategies and theories can provide in-depth insights which are difficult or impossible to achieve using other research methods.

Understanding the midwife respondents' experiences involves multiple sets of participation and observations. These include regular hospital visits, attending seminars, conference, developing the first midwifery research unit and working in the School of Nursing in *Hángzhōu* Normal University, China. The experiences of the first author as a midwife in China and the UK; and the second author, as a UK midwifery professor proved to be valuable in allowing us to see, understand and compare the development of Chinese midwifery with other cultures. Our own experiences as a midwife and social scientist were rather less important as a source of data but as a filter through which we interpreted and made sense of the material we collected. In this way the study is not only an account of what we have seen and perceived but also an explicit account of our inner experience or conflict as a midwife and social scientist. Therefore, the construction of the respondents' realities was taken as a miniature of the society they perceived but not necessarily an objective reflection of their reality (Haralambos & Holborn 2008: 812). However, the problem of trying to get to grips with what was happening remained as challenging and fascinating as ever.

Interviews

We, as a midwife and social scientist, interviewed Chinese midwives to collect first-hand materials. That offered us a way to ensure thorough immersion in the study. The interviews with midwives were carried out in Mandarin or local dialects. The oral history and verbal testimonies of experienced individuals were collected through semi-structured and unstructured interviews.

In this study, we carried out 38 semi-structured and unstructured interviews with 32 midwives, labour delivery room (LDR) nurses, midwife-obstetricians and six birth attendants from five villages, 12 cities and four municipalities directly under the central government across 13 provinces (Figure 2.1), from north to south, and central to south-west China.

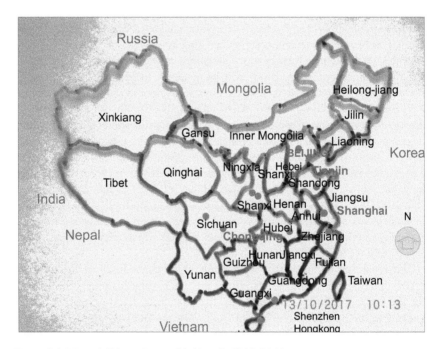

Figure 2.1 Map of China–places of fieldwork, 2007–2014

Note: Dots indicate the places where data were collected.

Comparison

A regional comparative qualitative approach (Barnard 2000:57) is adopted for this study to investigate the development of Chinese midwifery and experience of the midwives. This method is combined with the literature review, interviews and our experiences as a midwife in China and in Britain.

The social encounters with midwives interviewed and the interpretation of this process brought us to a question of 'regional diversities'. We do not see a straightforward link between those individual stories in the process of interpretation. Every story is unique in a sense. This does not prevent us from using the findings as an indication of midwives' beliefs and meanings of their social practice and conditions.

Another question is 'objectivity' and 'subjectivity'. We believe that we can be more 'objective' because we have taken all our 'subjectivities' into account. However, it is often when you think that you become more 'objective', you become more 'subjective' because in order to achieve that, people do not take into account themselves and some other things.

All the techniques, including literature review, participant observation, interview and comparison, help us interpret and understand the political, economic and social structure of Chinese midwifery, events and midwives, a mixture of available materials in order to show what it was and is like to be in the past and present. This wide-ranging approach attempts to move out of rigid categories, such as interviews, oral history, political history or social history. This rigorous and complex form helps us distinguish different roles, social status and pace of change in Chinese midwifery.

The interviews allow the authors to interact with the respondents to discover their meaningful interpretation and construction of their social reality. The participant observation captures the dynamic aspects of Chinese midwives' interaction with their clients and to check the understanding of the data from the other sources. The first-hand information fills the gaps in the existing Chinese midwifery literature. The recovered identity of Chinese midwives and the knowledge of the nature of their practice enable the authors to raise pertinent questions and to see the relationship of the identities, meanings and practice of Chinese midwifery. Their relationship is far from static but changing over time. A deeper understanding is developed through such a careful, constant study and analysis of empirical studies.

Data analysis

This cyclical thinking from the present to history and from history to the present is a very basic approach to this investigation. The tool of history–modernity dualism is believed to be able to improve understanding of the development of Chinese midwifery in terms of its social institutions and their management.

From a functional approach, the development of Chinese midwifery is related to our sociological understanding of modernity which led to the ways of thinking conducive to modernisation of midwifery. In particular, we anticipated it should be encouraged in order to achieve a greater sense of profession, self-reliance and independence (Harlambos & Holborn 2008).

The data analysis is undoubtedly guided by the values of the authors and the theoretical perspectives that influence our work most. The interpretation of the meanings held by the respondents is recovered or discovered from the actual interactions and their context. However, by being self-critical, we try to minimise the extent to which our own understanding distorts social reality and try to be more objective. By being explicit about our methods we hope other researchers will be able to evaluate our work.

Discussion

The decline of Chinese midwifery (Cheung et al. 2005a, 2005b, 2006a, b; Cheung 2009) has continued unchecked and the quality of maternity care has steadily deteriorated. The obstetric technologies were used extensively to the health workers' ends rather than the childbearing women's needs. This manipulation tends to obscure the relations between technology and the maternal function of women and to reinforce the medical control of technology and the bodies of women. Therefore, the study of history and modernity of Chinese midwifery concurrently can enable us to examine the process of changes in Chinese midwifery in the light of Chinese modernisation of health care which has brought about the dominance of the Western model of care and its value systems.

With a clear study orientation and the consideration of all the changes and dimensions in Chinese midwifery, the issue of its modernisation becomes complex and difficult to understand. In reality, we have seen some women with obstructed labour survive because of the power of obstetric technologies while others' bodies and lives have been controlled by the obstetric technology for social and financial reasons. Finally, we have realised the role that obstetric technologies have played in the medicalisation of childbirth. On one hand, this difficulty is because of a constant process of change of the profession in dramatically escalating the use of technology or 'industrialisation' in pursuit of efficiency and efficacy; on the other hand, the internalisation of these changes and dimensions reveals a deep-rooted problem in Chinese academics' understanding of modernity in health care provision, for example, the promotion of 100% hospitalisation of childbirth in China in the 21st century (CMoH et al. 2003). The present study delineates the developments and the relations between these periods by using the methods discussed earlier.

3 A holistic approach
Chinese midwifery before 1928

Introduction

Since the majority of the population of China lives on the mainland, the midwifery culture there is explored here as the basis for this book. The period covered in this chapter begins in 770 BCE (see Timeline) because the first Chinese medical book *Huángdì-nèijìng* (The Yellow Emperor's Classic of Internal Medicine) was believed to be written around that time (Wáng 762; Jia 1982; Furth 1999; Further Reading and Notes – Traditional Chinese medicine books pertinent to midwifery). It was the first textbook used in the imperial medical school and is still in widespread use as a classic textbook in some colleges or universities of Chinese medicine and beyond. Its modern version has no changes other than those in the punctuation. The book was an important source of Chinese philosophical thought and a key to the understanding of Chinese ancient curing and caring theory. The book was a collected work over time and consists of two sections: *Sùwèn* (Basic questions) and *Língshū* (Spiritual focus; *Wáng* 762). The former introduces the theoretical foundation of Chinese medicine and its diagnostic methods; the latter deals with acupuncture. The work has been regarded as a great source for Chinese medicine.

Qì, yīnyáng *and* wǔxīng *in traditional Chinese medicine*

In the previously mentioned books, *qì, yīnyáng* and *wǔxīng* (the Five Elements; Guide – Chinese glossary) were used as the principal medical theory to understand and explain the complex layers of interpretation of human diseases and the world (*Wáng* 762; Bynum & Bynum 2011).

Qì (air) is a hypothetical concept in the eye of modern science, which refers to air, blood and body fluids in human bodies. *Qì* is believed to be experienced and recognised as something of all reality, which is an invisible, dynamic and cosmic unity of the material world. It has the inherent property of *yīn* and *yáng* to reflect the simple concept of the unity of opposites; for example, illness is *yīn*, and health is *yáng*. This binary system forms a unity of *qì*, which is the root of all activities. *Qì* is believed to travel through the *jīngluò*, the network of channels through which vital energy circulates and along which key acupuncture points are distributed. *Jīngluò* consists of 12 *jīngmài* (channels) that connect with 12 organs: the lungs, large intestine, stomach, spleen, heart, small intestine, bladder, kidney, pericardium, gall bladder, liver and *sānjiāo* (triple-energiser, believed to be a metabolic mechanism; Guide – Chinese glossary). Each organ function corresponds to particular emotions and has a unique spirit with its own form and attributes. *Qì* is thus the key to the mysterious inter-mingling understanding of the universe at the levels of person, natural world and cosmos, an understanding of which is supposed to make possible a life of wholeness and integrity.

The concept of *yīn* and *yáng* explained the dialectical view of things or things; these relate to the existence of two internal/external opposing forces, growth and decline of transformation, coordination and balance. It is the development of the traditional Chinese philosophy, though rooted in the ontological monism in *qì* but more on the methodology of dialectic thinking.

Yīn, which originally means 'shady', is associated with the phenomenon of cold, winter, cloud, rain and darkness and symbolises femininity and negativity.

Yáng, which means 'sunny', is associated with heat, brightness and summer and symbolises masculinity and positivity.

The *yīnyáng* system has been used as a theoretical basis showing correlations between phenomena; it sometimes led to the discovery of meaningful causal con-nections, but they have also been used in a mystical manner (Topley 1976: 247). Many authors have addressed this natural philosophy in their works (Needham & Lu 1969; Topley 1970, 1978; Ahern1978a & 1978b; Anderson 1988: 188). How-ever, none of their research has studied the theory specifically.

The philosophy of *yīn* and *yáng* is used to analyse the contradictions of human health and disease and to clarify fundamental laws of life movement. A cosmic harmony is important for human well-being and the health of society. Any sign of imbalance of the *yīn* and *yáng* was expected to result in illness, thus offering a way of understanding ill health.

Wŭxīng is known as the Five Elements or Five Phases (Figure 3.1). It is a five-fold conceptual scheme that many traditional Chinese fields used to explain a wide array of phenomena from cosmic cycles to the interaction between human body and environment. The Five Elements are Metal (金*jīn*), Wood (木*mù*), Water (水*shuĭ*), Fire (火*huŏ*) and Earth (土*tŭ*). Each of them has a season, particular organs, emotions and senses (taste, smell, vision, touch and hearing) associated with it:

METAL: winter, lungs, and large intestine;
WOOD: spring, liver and gall bladder;
WATER: winter, kidneys and bladder;
FIRE: early summer, heart and small intestine;
EARTH: late summer, stomach and spleen.

The Five Elements are interrelated aspects of *qì* in the human body. An indi-vidual's health depends on the balance among them.

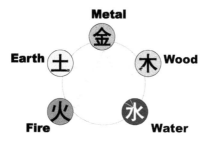

Figure 3.1 Wŭxīng, the Five Elements

In comparison, *qì* is more ontological in nature and intended to illustrate the unity of the universe and human life and death, while *yīnyáng* and *wŭxīng* are more methodological in feature. Illnesses are believed to be the result of unbalanced *qì*, disrupted interactions between the five elements, *yīnyáng* and other factors. Traditional Chinese medicine, therefore, often seeks to correct these imbalances by adjusting the circulation of *qì* using a variety of techniques including herbs, food therapy, moxibustion, acupuncture, exercises, *Qìgōng* (physical training regimens, and other martial arts) and others. This system is totally different from the biomedical approach in Western midwifery textbooks such a Mayes or Myles (Fraser & Cooper 2009). Its significance in Chinese medicine is similar to that of the Hippocratic Corpus in Greek medicine. The clinical skills are also similar, listening to, observing and palpating the pulse of patients carefully and treating them with sympathy, empathy and compassion.

The theory of *qì, yīnyáng* and *wŭxīng* is holistic and is unlike Western medicine in the sense that the focus of the latter is on organs, cells and molecules. Disease results from the malfunction of these units, and the patient, may sometimes slip from view. The focus of the *qì, yīnyáng* and *wŭxīng* is on the balance of the body and mind.

The theory of *qì, yīnyáng* and *wŭxīng* underscores the understanding of Chinese medicine that human beings function both physically and mentally. These interpretations are intertwined with nature. Though it may be difficult for people of other cultures to understand, it is fundamental to understanding traditional Chinese medicine.

Many Chinese visit their traditional doctors by their own choice. This does not necessarily mean they cannot afford the services of Western physicians. In fact, those physicians' services were often provided free of charge by churches in the past. People, who chose Chinese traditional medicine, have more confidence in it because they believed that traditional medicine had stood the test of time. This raises the question of whether traditional Chinese medicine could make the same claims to efficacy as Western medicine does. Neither the claims made by Western medicine nor by Chinese medicine, though, can stand up to the notion of 'science'. Traditional Chinese medicine has relied on a balance of the prehistoric mystic philosophical concept of *yīnyáng* and elements of superstition in diagnoses and treatments of diseases for centuries. However, people cannot deny its value when they are aware of its therapeutic effect, especially on chronic diseases. Western medicine tends to be controlled by modern technology in terms of too many operations and interventions.

The rise of biophysiological midwifery

The analysis of historical records suggests that 1928 was a point of departure, politically and professionally, from traditional practices in Chinese midwifery. This was when the first Midwives Rules, based on biophysiological medicine, were issued in 1928 by the Ministry of Health of the Nationalist Government (1928; Further Reading and Notes – Midwifery policies in China). Midwifery as a profession was thus changed gradually through organised educational programmes, regulations of midwifery practice, and education throughout urban and some rural areas in China. Childbirth and midwives were shifted gradually from home to hospital with the development of biophysiological medicine, education of physicians and new childbirth technologies.

In reality there is a wealth of evidence that the diffusion of European medicine into China, which impacted on midwifery practice, could be seen as having started in 1838 when a Medical Missionary Society was established (Chang 2003: 152). In 1909 a Christian Missionary's Nurses' Association of China (CMNAC) was set up (see Chapter 3, Simpson 1929: 138). It issued qualifications to nurses in China after three years of training and to midwives after at least a further year of training before they began practice. Midwifery as an organised profession in China did not officially exist before 1928. Midwives were certainly used, but not necessarily appreciated, by the rulers. They were either summoned or promoted by the imperial courts to provide helping hands to bring forth the imperial successors. But as an agrarian empire, China did not seem to have the society for a large-scale and organised midwifery profession. What we know was that most villages or neighbourhoods used family-inherited and part-time practices. As in many other human societies, births were very important social events in Chinese societies.

Midwives were expected to be old and experienced and were often appreciated and respected in individual cases. But they were generally downgraded in terms of their professional significance. That could be expected in view of the patriarchal ideology prevailing in central China since the beginning of its history. China had had some contact since the *Qín* Dynasty (秦; see Timeline) with other kingdoms, societies, countries, or tribes in central, south, and south-east Asia; in the Middle East; in south-eastern Europe; and in Africa. Such contact was mostly through trade and religion, but it was not on such a scale as to influence midwifery practice until the late 19th century.

The immediate concerns of Chinese rulers from very early times were to defend their borders and control their country. This is reflected on its border-building work, the Great Wall. There were many periods when the rulers took the view that the rest of the world was poor and backward with little to offer. The door to business and trade was blocked to them. Literacy was the privilege of the elite, whose education had been centred on breadth and stability. The patriarchal ideology barred women from education because their place was considered to be diligence rather than creativity. Confucius's teaching influenced the thoughts and behaviour of many Chinese. Prescriptive in nature, Confucius (551–479 BCE) considered that everyone should occupy a social place in an orderly world, some were 'higher', such as rulers, parents and husbands; others were 'lower', for example, subjects, children and wives. No matter what their social status was, everyone was bound together in ties of mutual duty and respect. When these bonds were broken, the stability of the society was threatened.

China was more united by a written language and culture than it was by political structure. A written Chinese script is difficult to learn as it is not necessarily linked to the sound of language. It can certainly facilitate communication with others and provides a bond for people of different languages and dialects. That is why China has retained a unity of culture, though it has been politically divided in history and the present. *Hàn* (205 BCE–220 CE; see Timeline), *Táng* (618–907 CE) and *Sòng* (960–1279 CE) were the most powerful dynasties. During these periods, trade flourished and China grew prosperous, with an efficient administration, extensive roads and the Great Canal, which linked *Běijīng* with *Hángzhōu*. Huge irrigation projects provided food for the growing population in an increasing number of large towns and cities. The change in lifestyle brought a change in scholarship, belief systems, trade along the 'Silk Road', and inventions such as paper, printing, casting of iron, magnetic compasses and gunpowder. Cliff-side carvings and cave paintings in the *Sòng* dynasty give glimpses of what happened during that time. Settled agriculture brought with it a new emphasis on birth and fertility which were symbolised by the carvings in *Dàzú*. The artefacts during this period are discussed in Chapter 9.

Traditional midwifery as an occupation was respectable before the *Sòng* dynasty (960–1279 CE; Leung 2000) but descended to a nadir by the *Míng* dynasty (1368–1644 CE) as it was realised that maternity care requires more than just compassion. During the early *Qīng* dynasty (1616–1911 CE), Europeans sailed the seven seas in search of goods to trade and new lands to conquer. Colonies were built and expanded. By the end of the 17th century, only Oceania remained undiscovered by the Europeans. However, trade with Western nations was not permitted, as the emperor considered his country was rich enough and did not need anything from the west. Only after the two Opium Wars (1839–1842, 1856–1860 CE) with Britain, and later France, did the control of the *Qīng* Dynasty began to decline. Reluctantly, China had to open its doors to European powers. Western medicine, focusing on the physical human body, organs, tissues, cells and molecules, eventually reached China in the early 18th century when some missionaries trained in medicine began to extend their activities to Chinese patients in China (Halde 1738; Veith 1949: 1). After the inauguration of the Medical Missionary Society in China in 1838 (Li & Guo 2009: 3), the scope of Western medicine increased rapidly. However, Chinese midwifery was little influenced by this development and remained insignificant.

The organised biomedical education of midwifery and midwives' organisations started much earlier in Taiwan Province. The earliest record of biophysiological midwives there dates back to 1907 during the Japanese occupation (Chiou & Chou 2006). It was five years after English midwives' legislation. After that, the Midwives Registration Ordinance, which is now known as the Midwives Council of Hong Kong (MCOHK 2014) was first enacted in 1910. In mainland China, the Nurses' Association of China (NAC) was established in 1909 (Li & Guo 2009) by six foreign nurses and three doctors (Simpson 1923; Chang 2003: 155), under a Christian missionary. The first draft of the Midwives Rules by the Chinese government was not published until 1928. In the following year, the first state recognised midwifery school was officially set up in *Běijīng* (Liu 2005).

Before the introduction of Western European medicine into China, traditional midwives learned their craft through apprenticeship and tradition. They were not educated about scientific advances, such as preventing infection. Around this time, the criticism from Chinese medicine-men was against midwives' illiteracy, which might lead to poor outcomes for mothers and babies. The widespread criticisms prompted the establishment of the first Midwives Rules in 1928 and midwifery school in 1929. It aimed to incorporate the necessary medical training into midwifery's traditional approach to pregnancy and labour. The revolution of thinking and industrialisation became the generally accepted features in the 1920s and 1930s.

We will now look more closely at six aspects of the development of midwifery through history.

Traditional midwifery

Traditional midwifery before 1928 had a different approach to the understanding of childbearing, childbirth and child-rearing. It was influenced by the traditional concepts of *qì, yīnyáng* and *wǔxíng* which could be observed from the Yellow Emperor's Classic of Internal Medicine (*Wáng* 762; Topley 1970: 423, 1978: 128; Unschuld 1985). Similar to traditional Chinese medicine but less complicated, any disturbance of the balance of *yīn* and *yáng* would result in disease. Thus, the *yīnyáng* system has been used to classify all aspects of childbearing, from conception to postnatal care and from daily activities to diet (Cheung 1996a, 1996b, 1997; Cheung et al. 2006a). Obedience to the laws of *yīnyáng* means life; disobedience means death. *Yīnyáng* is perceived as the most basic division of the cosmos in traditional Chinese thought (*Wáng* 762: 31), dualism operating within every entity.

The focus of this system during childbearing is on the balance of mind, body, spirit and soul as a whole rather than on specific parts or aspects of a woman's body. This requires women to keep harmony within the family, maintain lifestyle equilibrium and carry out fetal education during pregnancy to facilitate their health and that of their foetus. It is, therefore, termed a holistic approach here to differentiate it from biomedical midwifery. As most traditional midwives were illiterate (Lee 2008: 127), *yīnyáng* was understood as 'hot' and 'cool' by the people in southern China and 'fire' and 'cold' in the north. Hence, the traditional medical theory of *qì*, *yīnyáng* and *wǔxīng w*as simplified by laypeople to a system of *yīn and yáng* that they could understand. This philosophical, conceptual dualism between mind and body forms the basis of Chinese thought and has reflected the development of the rationality of traditional Chinese medicine in the works of *Lǐ Shízhēn*, an ancient Chinese herbalist (*Lǐ* 1596: 26–8; Guide – Chinese glossary). This is not because they are scientific or philosophical but because of their practicality and a firm belief in their great value.

The practitioners of this system were termed traditional midwives in this study. They were a complicated social group without biomedical training, being an 'occupation' or 'trade', albeit lower in the social hierarchy. The appellation (Guide – Chinese glossary) applied to these maternity service providers in Chinese history revealed complicated social facts about them: that they had internal hierarchies and that they had regional as well as social variations. Traditional midwives were first known as 'great aunt' or 'granny' respectfully and, less respectfully, as *zhuòpó* (坐婆), *kānchǎn* (看产), *kǎnshēngrén*（看生人）, or *shōushēngzhīfù* (收生之妇; Guide – Chinese glossary). Later in the 14th century, when female occupations were categorised, they became *wěnpó*（稳婆）or *chǎnpó*（产婆） and then *jiēshēngpó*（接生婆） in the early 20th century (Lee 1999, 2005; Leung 2000; Harris et al. 2009a).

Normally traditional midwives were married or widowed women. They had grown-up families and usually were over 40 and respected locally (*Chén* 1237). This can be clearly observed from the fact that the average age of the 30 students in the first recruitment of the *Běipíng* Birth Attendant School in *Běijīng* in 1928 was 54 years old (CCTV 2005). Their age, reputation and their personal experience in childbirth were deemed to give them sufficient qualifications for their job (Tew 1998; Leung 2000; Lee 2003, 2005). The situation of Chinese midwives was similar to that of the midwives in ancient Athens, who, by law, were required to have had children themselves because personal experience was the most important qualification (Radcliff 1967).

Traditional midwives were usually illiterate and had no medical training. They learnt their skills from personal experience and through looking after their own family, apprenticeship or knowledge inherited from older generations (Tew 1998; Leung 2000; Lee 2003). This is further discussed in Chapters 9 and 10. Childbearing was considered women's business and had always been the preserve of women, traditionally providing a livelihood for the wife and the widow. It was traditional midwives who came to women in labour and who assisted them in giving birth. The more births they attended, the more experienced they became, and the more their services were sought.

Sometimes, when labour complications occurred, such as malpresentation, obstruction and retained placenta and haemorrhage, medicine-men were called in to give some advice, but they were barred from the birthing room (Furth 1987; Lee 2003).

'Good' traditional midwives were considered old, kind and honest, and they had a reputation for their skills. The majority of them remained in and served their own communities (*Chén* 1237; *Fù* 1425; Furth 1987). The better ones were selected by their local regional administration officers to be 'woman doctors' or women healers (女医 *nǚyī*, 为医 *wéiyī*) to serve the royal family in the Imperial Palace (Lee 2008: 249). They were also called *wěnpó* in their communities. Their practice was heavily influenced by astrology, ancestry, witchcraft or demonology, and difficult labours were attributed to these influences. When midwives attended births, some would choose a south facing direction for the labour room and an auspicious time (Lee 2008). They sometimes invited astrologers, or fortune tellers to cast a horoscope for the newborn and the mother, as happened in Europe before the 20th century (Ehrenreich & English 1973; Ehrenreich 1976; Oakley & Houd, 1990: 21).

However, Chinese midwives did not leave us many of their stories either because of their illiteracy (Lee 2003) or because Chinese history focused on the incessant struggle between central power and local interests (Schurmann & Schell 1967a, b, c). Their experience and knowledge about birthing and birth assistance were passed on within their family from one generation of women to another. As in the West, Chinese historical records largely neglect the life of common people, particularly the life of women and traditional midwives. We know them only through passing remarks made by some Chinese literati, medicine-men, historians and journalists.

Traditional childbirth and midwifery in China have been mentioned by some sinologists and Chinese historians (Ahern 1978a, b; Wolf 1978; Lee 2008). They have explored the relevant terms, concepts and practices in childbirth from 206 BCE to 1279 CE. The practice of '*giving birth on grass*' (下地坐草) in the *Suí* and the *Táng* dynasties was reported by Lee (1999, 2003, 2008) and Leung (2000); 'sitting on a straw mat to give birth' (坐蓐分娩) in *Hángzhōu* in the early 20th century (Hu 1922a: 167). According to *Zhēn Zhìyà* and *Fù Wéikāng* about 90 different medical history books have been published and distributed (*Zhēn & Fù* 1991: 467), but the history of midwifery has been neglected.

Some American historians and anthropologists have given attention to the concept of pregnancy and birth in Chinese culture (Furth 1987). As childbirth had been the province of female practitioners, the studies of China by the early predominantly male anthropologists, explorers and missionaries were merely on kinship, religions, customs, family, gender, society, medicine and food but not childbirth or midwifery (Croll 1985a, b, 1995; Ahern 1978a, b, c; Wolf 1978).

However, childbirth and female reproductive disorders had long been recognised in Chinese medicine. Women were perceived, as in other parts of the world (Wajcman 1993: 67), as frail and prone to physical and mental disease by *Chén Zìmíng* in his book *Fùrén dàquán Liáng fāng* written in 1237, the first comprehensive book on midwifery and gynaecology in Chinese traditional medicine. In addition, being able to produce sons was crucial, so women's bodies were a prime object of medical attention and many Chinese medical works discussed them.

Separation of *fùkē* (medicine for women) from Chinese medicine

Before 256 BCE the *yīnyáng* theory of Chinese medicine, midwifery and other categories were all the same (Fu 1982: 42–5). Curing and healing had been achieved through tackling the balance of *yīn* and *yáng* of the body and symptoms with herbal treatments, diets, fluid intake and rest. The earliest evidence of the discussion of *fùkē* was *Bèijí-qiānjīn yàofāng* (Further Reading and Notes – Traditional Chinese medicine books pertinent to midwifery) written by *Sūn sīmiǎo* in 652 CE. *Fùkē*, medicine for women, or midwifery and gynaecology in modern terms, was finally separated from traditional Chinese medicine by the appearance of another two books: *Jīng-xiào-chǎn-bǎo* (Further Reading and Notes – Traditional Chinese medicine books pertinent to midwifery) by *Zǎn Yīn* in 847 and *Chǎn-yù-bǎo-qīng-fāng* (Further Reading and Notes – Traditional Chinese medicine books pertinent to midwifery) by *Guō Qīzhōng* in 1109, though they were quite simple (Liang 1983).

Midwifery and gynaecology became firmly established as independent subjects following the appearance of *Fùrén dàquán fāng* (Further Reading and Notes – Traditional Chinese medicine books pertinent to midwifery). It was written in 1237 by *Chén Zìmíng* (1237) and is the first comprehensive book on Chinese midwifery and gynaecology.

There are 24 chapters in the book dealing mainly with eight topics: menstruation, pregnancy disorders, conception, 'foetal education', pregnancy, sitting in for the month, difficult labour and postnatal care (Chen 1237). His book was a good example of an 'eclectic' medical system (Furth 1987: 8), which was based on his own and others' accumulated clinical experience; it drew on the belief in the symbolic significance of women's reproduction and a social model of power and weakness. In Chen's book, women were presented, on one hand, as powerful because they could give birth to babies, the heir of the family. On the other hand, they were weak because their illness was 10 times more difficult to treat than men and polluting in the form of menstruation and lochia, which is further discussed in this chapter and Chapter 9. These images became more obvious, especially in the discussion of menstruation, fetal education and sitting in for the month. His book made him the first comprehensive dominant medicine-man for women's diseases in Chinese history.

Fùrén dàquán fāng illustrates the changes made in Chinese midwifery during that period. The changes made were direct responses to their immediate environment and the development of Chinese medicine and changes in ideology. The records made were a matter of handed-down knowledge, experience and word of mouth. Although the general approach is said to be holistic, the author's attitude towards women's diseases is quite masculine and medically orientated in that he identified women's bodies as the source of many health problems.

The imperial Chinese medical school

By 443 CE, China had its first socially organised medical education, offered in the imperial palace (Gao 1982: 135–40). This was known as the imperial medical school which was named differently in different time periods. It was '*tàiyīshǔ*' (太医署) in the *Táng* dynasty (618–907 CE), '*tàiyījú*' (太医局) in the *Sòng* dynasty (960–1279 CE), '*tàiyīyuàn*' (太医院) in the *Yuán* (Mongol) dynasty (1206–1368 CE; see Timeline; Guide – Chinese glossary). There was no clear indication of the students' gender in this school. However, a collection of Japanese court regulations, *Seiji yōyaku*, reported a record of 30 medicine-women aged between 15 and 25 selected from official slaves to the palace, which was considered to be a duplicate practice of the Chinese *Táng* dynasty (618–907 CE; Lee 2003: 18–20). These student 'medicine-women' were instructed orally about calming the foetus, helping in childbirth, nursing wounds, acupuncture and moxibustion. Those who passed the examinations would be recruited into the imperial court and those who failed would be dismissed. The length of their study was seven years, while the male medical students studied for two to seven years depending on their subject (Gao 1982: 138).

In Chinese history, the imperial palace was the only place known to train medicine-men and -women officially. Outside it, there were masses of apprentices of self-trained healers and traditional midwives. There were neither any organised trade guilds, like the barber-surgeons in the UK (Donnison 1988; Tew 1998), nor any licensing laws enforcing any medical practices. Therefore, China was awash with medicine-men, medicine-women, shaman and healers of all kinds before the 19th century (Leung 2000; Lee 2003). Obviously, the imperial medical examination system simply could not or would not include those practitioners who provided services to ordinary people or provide them with professional training and education.

Schools of medicine in the *Sòng* and *Yuán* dynasties stressed preventive care, while schools in the *Míng* and *Qīng* dynasties emphasised convalescence and regulation of diet (Watt 2004: 68). Home remained the base for the patient's care, even after Chinese medicine adopted the Western hospital system in the late 20th century and professional nursing became part of that care.

Nurses' Association of China

Modern nursing in China was of recent origin and was started by Missionary doctors and nurses. As a missionary nurse, Miss Simpson (1923: 138) stated in her 1923 report in the *British Journal of Nursing* that China 'is the one country in the world where Christian nurses were free to establish ideals and carry them to a full fruition unhampered'. In just 10 years' time, the scattered groups of missionary nurses were organised, set up the Nurses' Association of China (NAC) in 1909 and prepared a programme for the standard curriculum, registration of schools, national examinations and diploma. According to its rules, only a nurse after having secured the association's diploma (three years), she may enter for the normal midwifery diploma (one year), and after she holds that she may still sit for the diploma in operative midwifery (Simpson 1913, 1923: 139).

The NAC development is the result of colonisation of China by Westerners. According to Halde (1738), Western medicine did not reach China until the early 18th century when Jesuits who had been trained in medicine extended their activities to Chinese patients. The first full-time missionary doctor Peter Parker came to *Guǎngzhōu* in 1834 (Chang 2003: 152). He opened the first ophthalmic hospital in the following year (Simpson 1923: 138–9; Chang 2003: 152; Li & Guo 2009). The Medical Missionary Society was established in *Guǎngzhōu* by missionaries on 21 February 1838. The first job of the society was to support the ophthalmic hospital run by Dr Peter Parker and then introduced Western medicine into China, as medicine could assist spreading Christianity (Veith 1949; Lǐ & Guo 2009: 3). From then on, biomedicine in China consolidated steadily.

After the two Opium Wars of 1839–1842 and 1856–1860 (Schurmann & Schell 1967a) China had to open its ports by the humiliatingly unequal Treaties of Nanking (*Nánjīng* 南京) and Tientsin (*Tiānjīn* 天津) to trading, owning property and spreading faith in China. These ports were Canton (*Guǎngdōng* 广东), Amoy (*Xiàmén* 厦门), *Fúzhōu, Wēnzhōu, Níngbō* and *Shànghǎi* (Stowell 1954). Foreigners with passports were allowed to travel in the interior and Christian missionary activities were permitted. As well as trading and other privileges, foreigners living in treaty ports were not subject to Chinese law. Chinese people resented these privileges, and many revolutionary efforts were directed against foreigners. Despite all this, many missionary hospitals were set up in major cities of China. There were more than 50 hospitals by 1890 (Li & Guo 2009), and gradually, missionary hospitals had reached every part of China and the hospitals had to confront an acute shortage of nurses because China, then, did not have this profession.

The first Christian nurse to come to China was Miss Elizabeth McKechnie from the US. She arrived at *Shànghǎi* in 1884. Twenty-five years later, Christian nurses were dispersed all over and always working there as nurse teachers and superintendents. When Cora E. Simpson (信宝珠, US) came to Foochow (*Fúzhōu*), China, in 1907, she was told that China did not need and was not ready for nurses as patients had always been cared by their family members and friends. After a day in the hospital and a few visits out into the homes, she saw the country in desperate need of nurses. She wrote in 1908 to Dr PB Cousland (高士兰, US) of *Shànghǎi*, the president of the China Medical Association, asking about organising nurses' work in China. Her letter and the reply to her request were put into a leaflet form and sent out in the *China Medical Journal* of that year as a call to nurses to form an association.

The NAC was thus organised and established despite unimaginable demands and difficulties on 1909 with Mrs. C.M. Hart (赫特, Canadian, sent by US missionaries) of *Wúhú* (芜湖) as the first president, Ms. M. Ogden (奥格登) as vice president and Miss M.T. Henderson (亨德森, UK) of Wusih (*Wúxī* 无锡) as the secretary. The other six participants of the inaugural meeting in Kuling (*Gǔlǐng* 牯岭), *Jiāngxī* Province were Dr PB Cousland, Dr Lucy A. Gaynor (盖纳, US) of

Nanking (*Nánjīng* 南京), Dr Mary Hannah Fulton (富尔顿, US) of Kwangtung (*Guǎngdōng*), Ms Alice Clark (克拉克, US) of *Shànghǎi* and Ms. N.D. Gage (盖仪贞, US) and Ms. L.A. Batty (贝孟雅, UK) of *Hànkǒu* (Simpson 1923: 138–9; Li & Guo 2009: 9–12; Li & Guo 2009: 10).

The NAC development opened a new world and, maybe unintentionally, created new Chinese words for nurses (*hùshì* 护士) and midwives (*zhù-chǎn-nǚ-shì* 助产女士, nowadays *zhù-chǎn-shì* 助产士, as the character representing females was dropped). In the past China did not have a word for nurses (*hùshì* 护士), even less a profession or an organised professional body. The closest equivalent to the title was the word *kānhù* (看护, orderly in charge of care).

The new imported biomedical practices led eventually to a bill for a provisional ban on birth attendants in 1913 issued by the Department of the Capital Police of the *Běiyáng* government (1912–28) of the Republic of China (1911–date; DCPBGC 1913). In reality, this ban was never implementable for three reasons. First, the government was corrupt and incompetent. Second, the policy did not give any consideration to the acute shortage of trained health workers at that time and the impact of this ban on the lives of women and families. Third, even if the policy-makers had time, there was not enough time to train appropriate competent staff for the needs of the country to take over the workload of 'banned' birth attendants.

Although this ban remained, traditional birth attendants continued to practise as usual even up to today, especially in rural and remote areas.

Lay and formal care: blurred boundaries

In China at that time, lay and biomedical care was often distinguished by the place where the care happened. The formal biomedical care usually took place in hospitals, with informal care at home. Meanwhile, the traditional Chinese medical practitioners of all kinds continued to practise medicine, mainly on a part-time basis, and learned by experience. The legitimacy of caring and healing was earned by the approval of the community who received the service. It can be imagined that the Chinese communities were very pragmatic towards these services. Disputes after the services must have been handled either through payments, social position, personal relations, public opinion or according to the decrees of local magistrates.

With the arrival of Western medicine, and the Euro-American style of maternity care, the practice of midwifery in China was transformed. Care given at home was moved to newly built hospitals or provided by Western obstetricians. Modern hospitals laid stress on anatomy, empirical physiological and biological learning and formal training. Full-time employment in medicine, with certification institutions and responsibility systems in place, was no longer only to serve the rulers but was intended to serve the whole society. Such organised public medical care provision, to which midwifery services were attached, had never existed before in China. It can be said that, as in other spheres of life, medicine and medical care had been industrialised, as practices became increasingly specialised and professionalised.

During the period between about 1910 and 1930, one foreign-trained nurse was all any hospital could boast. Formal midwifery training was only possible at hospitals in big cities which had been long established and large enough to be able to take pupil midwives. Only those nurses who were well known enough would be called out for normal cases, and the doctor in charge was only called out for abnormal cases. These difficult cases sometimes followed traditional birth attendants having done their best and their worst.

If a woman in a major city was persuaded to give birth in hospital, she was obliged to stay in hospital for a month after the birth; this was because her family would not allow her home because of their concerns about the polluting effects of birth blood (lochia, discussed in the next section). Additionally, they feared that the new mother might have contact with cold and/or wind which might endanger her health and, more important, that of her newborn baby.

The legacy of the traditional practices, plus the availability and management of modern public resources within the state power, resulted in the differentiation between professional care, which may be termed 'formal care', on one hand, and the lay, or 'informal care', on the other. Women throughout recorded history have helped their neighbours to give birth, using their own experience as mothers. They learned what to do by doing and personal experience. They were more available in slums than medicine-men. Women practitioners' midwifery skills were gained mainly on an occasional basis through their own experiences of giving birth, learning from others and supporting neighbours, friends or relatives during childbirth. The regulation and control of these practitioners were inconsistent and were mainly by word of mouth or through social sanctions.

The professionalisation of medicine-men, nurses and traditional midwives for the general public did not take place until the appearance of the first public medical university in 1898 in *Běijīng* (*Peking* University 2017). The first private missionary midwifery school, opened in 1900, registered with the NAC in 1918 as *Pútián* St Luke's School of Midwifery (Wei 2011: 40) and then came the first national midwifery school in Beijing in 1928. These were milestones in providing a standardised institutional training and established the criteria for certifying nursing and midwifery practitioners.

A midwife's duty, no matter whether traditional care or modern professional care, continued through all stages of pregnancy, birth and after the birth as she attended the baby, mother and family. The boundary between formal and informal midwifery care was blurred.

Skills and status

The traditional idea that women were not suitable to practise general medicine does not mean that women were excluded from attending childbirth in China. No evidence has been found to suggest women were prohibited from practising midwifery before 1928. The Chinese recognised the fact that midwives' knowledge was rooted in their being women. Midwifery practice was traditionally open to any woman who could demonstrate healing skills (Unschuld 1985; Lee 2008), although Dàoist and Buddhist monks and nuns were banned in 653 CE by the imperial palace from practising medicine and shamanistic healing (Lee 2003).

However, a patriarchal Chinese society did not think highly of women's intelligence as women were looked on as caretakers of the home and family. This is largely due to their greater responsibility for children and dependent care and household tasks. Women were believed to be weaker biologically than men in Chinese culture because of their three types of polluting blood: flowing blood, menstrual blood and birth blood (Ahern 1978c). Anyone who had contact with menstrual blood and lochia would be considered polluted, barred from worshipping the gods, and render any medicine ineffective. So midwives were not allowed to be present during the administration of medicines (Ahern 1978c; Lee 2003). The concept of pollution metaphorically was an expression and reflection on women or midwives' social role and their social activities.

The social status of traditional midwives was humble and low because of Confucius's teaching of *sāncóng side* (see Guide – Chinese glossary) for women. The social exclusion of women from literacy kept them from generating and incorporating new knowledge of their contemporary community and from any systematic study about them and the further development of midwives' practices. This could be observed further from the occupational cliché, *sāngū liùpó* (see Guide – Chinese glossary) which was used to address working women in all walks of life from 1300 and 1400 CE and discussed by many sociologists and anthropologists (Furth 1987; Lee 1999; Leung 2000). Midwives were the lowest of the occupational groups (see Chapter 8). Nevertheless, their job rendered them powerful because birthing was a rite of passage for women in their family building and midwives, as women's supporters and childbirth facilitators, constituted part of the culture.

The Chinese *Hàn–Táng* (206 BCE–907 CE) historian Professor Lee (1996: 573) argues that midwifery has been an occupation since the *Hàn* dynasty (206 BCE–220 CE). This may have been a statement based strictly on written evidence. One can easily argue that midwifery is one of the most ancient occupations since the beginning of humanity (Donnison 1988). The first birth attendants were, as stated previously, probably the labouring woman's self-taught female relatives or friends. Their skills must have been obtained through their personal experience, observation and daily reiterated discourses. Such speculation on the beginning of midwifery has also been related to Western midwifery (Radcliff 1967; Ehrenreich 1976; Towler & Bramall 1986; Donnison 1988; Tew, 1998).

Birth attendants from 960 to 1911 were considered to be professionals by Leung (2000) and Furth (1987), though an organised professional structure was absent from the traditional Chinese medical system. A question which arises is, 'What are the differences between "professionals then" and the "professionals now"?' This is further discussed in Chapter 5.

Changes and chances

Since the early 20th-century Western medicine has transformed the Chinese perception of midwifery. The development of technology focused on understanding causes, care and cures. Finding a way forward for midwifery in China was complicated by the cultural diversity of the country. Changes were constantly creating opportunities in trade and the crafts and new environments. At the same time, traditional midwives needed to confront change and the unknown. Some of these developments have been well documented.

Shèngjīng Hospital in *Shěnyáng*, northern China, was one of the missionary hospitals established in 1883 by a Scottish missionary Dr Dugald Christie (SHOCM 2007), and a Women's Hospital (see Guide – Chinese glossary) was subsequently built by him in 1894. There were two female doctors from Europe, two Chinese medicine-women and some female students working in the hospital in 1897. A maternity unit was established in 1916 and expanded into a four-storey hospital in 1930 when outpatients presenting at the hospital reached 99,487. The number of births in the first year reached 721, including 481 'difficult' labours (*Wáng* et al. 1983: 3288–9) This suggests that home births were more prevalent. Women gave birth in the hospital only when labour was difficult. The running costs of the hospital was funded by donations from local communities and British churches.

Another development was Peking Union Medical College (PUMC), 'cradle of modern medicine in China' (Andrews & Bullock 2014), which was founded in 1917 by the Rockefeller Foundation (PUMC 2018). Many key clinical specialties in China were founded by its faculty and graduates. The Nursing School of the PUMC was established in 1920 and has been a national teaching and research centre ever since. The PUMC Department of 'Social Services' was established in 1921 (*Yáng* 2006: 112) and antenatal check-ups were introduced by the public health department. The rise of biomedicine and modern midwifery progressed and modern Chinese midwifery evolved and was strengthened by these new developments.

Traditional midwives, *shōushōng lǎolao* (收生姥姥) or birth attendants continued to visit the pregnant women to get to know the clients' house before the onset of labour and attended the birth. They were usually illiterate and middle-aged. They may have learned their skills from their personal birthing experience and through looking after their own family. Alternatively, they inherited their skills from their mothers or grandmothers. They attended childbirth and, more important, worked as ritual specialists (*Yáng* 2006: 129), especially on day 3 for the baby bath in *Běijīng*. Such a background made it difficult for them to assert the value of their expertise and to define the boundaries of the profession.

Chinese midwives observed traditional practices, including explaining the meaning of and arranging the rituals associated with birth (*Yáng* 2006: 129–33). As in other societies, having a baby in a Chinese society was not simply human reproduction. It had bestowed a new role on the birthing woman as a social being, that is becoming a mother. For the newborns, birth initiated their life and existence in society. Anthropology terms this 'a rite of passage' in the life cycle of humankind (van Gennep 1909). Giving birth and being born featured rites in human lives. These rites created social solidarity, holding the community together. The child was not just physically separated from the mother but also socially and spiritually created and accepted. This was the occasion for a midwife to display her skills and even use spells as if she was controlling events and governing natural or supernatural forces. The Chinese traditional midwives had to face religious sanction as well, for example, when they encountered illegitimate births or abortion. In the traditional Chinese birthing culture, there were symbolic logic and meanings constituting the cosmos of birth and explaining the social relations between the newborn and their family networks (Lee 2008: 76–96, 137–201), which must have been known to the midwives. In cases of illegitimacy or abortion, explanations were applied by the midwifery services, so midwives were crucial, not only for resolving problems associated with births but also in maintaining social order,

Discussion

Much of the material in this chapter and in some other parts of the book just happen to have survived from the messy lives which midwives lived. Additionally, they have not been treated as historically significant. It is our intention, through the medium of this book, to leave a record for posterity and for education in Chinese midwifery. These are, nevertheless, sources open for historical interpretation. They can help us to reinterpret and reconstruct the lives, work and history of Chinese midwives for the future development of Chinese midwifery. The historical account of their legacy would provide a vivid sense of midwifery's importance and its professional development. However, we also need to be able to appreciate, apart from the richness of diversity, the limitations of the material and the complexity of the evidence.

This chapter explains why the development of Chinese midwifery was divided into two stages: before and after 1928. It has also presented the system of *qì*, *yīnyáng* and *wǔxīng* in relation to health, childbirth and some aspects of traditional Chinese midwifery. The issues of the skills and status of traditional midwives were discussed and their job was considered more appropriately as an occupation or trade rather than 'profession' during this early period in terms of the organisational structure of Chinese midwifery. Whether the history of Chinese midwifery is best understood as a sequence of events, a succession of time frames, a system of ideas, a set of parallel regional traditions or a process of constant change are further discussed in the remaining chapters in Part I.

4 Chinese midwifery in the 20th century

Highs and lows

A symbolic turning point for Chinese midwifery occurred in 1928 when the first draft of the biomedical Midwives Rules was published in July 1928. This was a crucial aspect of the regulation of midwifery, which is an example of the growth of hierarchies of bureaucrats in maternity care of modern China. The concept of 'modern' is intellectually complex in the science of society. To simplify, it may simply denote radical social and cultural changes as in contrast to that of the past. This is a rough stand we take in the present book. Thus, 1928 is seen as when an important change took place in midwifery in China, when a qualification verification rule was adopted in a new practice model (along the line of the new European concept of medicine). On the other hand, 1993 signified the profession's downfall because midwifery education was formally discontinued in the metropolises. By 1996, the profession was collapsing, with midwives being replaced by doulas.

Marking the beginning of Chinese midwifery as a profession, 1928 saw the enactment of the first Midwives Rules into law in China (Further Reading and Notes – Midwifery policies in China, Table 3.1). This positive development represents the high-water mark in the history of Chinese midwifery. In 1996, because the government believed that midwifery was backward, it discontinued education and employment in the urban health system in the name of 'modernisation'. The midwifery workforce was then transformed into nurses, doulas or doctors and disappeared completely from the formal health system. Such transformation, maintained by recurrent misunderstandings and stipulations of health policies, has increased and not decreased with the lapse of time. These changes have been reinforced by attempts to modernise agriculture, industry, national defence and science and technology.

This chapter addresses Chinese midwifery from 1928 to 1996, demonstrating the rise and eventual dismantling of Chinese midwifery. It further explores Chinese midwifery's ups and downs, their schools, midwives' rules and standards, work, associations, social standing and place in public life during this period.

The rise of Chinese midwifery – the Midwives Rules and standards

Following the establishment of Medical Missionary Society in China in 1838, the impact of Western medicine increased swiftly despite resistance from Chinese medicine (Veith 1949: 1; Chang 2003: 152). At the start of the 19th century, there was an intellectual surge in urban areas to learn more about Western medicine (Schurmann & Schell 1967a). Many reasonably sized hospitals with maternity units and medical schools were established in the major cities of China along the south-east coast by Western medically trained missionaries. Later hospitals were established by Chinese medical practitioners after returning from postgraduate studies abroad. Western practices gradually penetrated throughout China. However, rural areas remained relatively unaffected.

Since the establishment of the Nurses' Association of China (NAC) in 1909, registration of schools, national examinations and diplomas had developed steadily and healthily. The first registration system of Chinese midwives was created after Midwives Rules were eventually written and published by the Chinese Ministry of Health (CMoH) in July 1928 (CMoH 1928). The rules were amended in May 1929, requiring all midwives to pass a written and a clinical examination. China followed Western countries (Donnison 1988; Marland 1993), gradually introducing registration systems for doctors, midwives and nurses, primarily to control the quality of the health services and, supposedly, to safeguard public health and well-being. One could no longer call oneself a midwife based on self-training and apprenticeship. The midwife had to be reasonably well educated and be accountable for her practice to the public.

Enactment of the 1928 Midwives Rules was an important landmark for Chinese midwifery because it entered the public domain and became a government-endorsed profession. It meant the title of midwife became protected by law for the first time; additionally, the relationship between educated midwives and better outcomes for women and their babies was, effectively, acknowledged (Shao 1934). It also meant that midwives who passed the examinations, if they wished, could continue to practise independently with the state's approval.

Tasks of the Midwives Rules

The Midwives Rules in China share historical roots and run parallel with events happening in the UK, as the Chinese development of medicine, nursing and midwifery was closely linked with Western missionaries and the Medical Missionary Society.

The key tasks of the Rules in China were to

- establish and maintain a record of registered midwives,
- establish standards of midwifery care to be met by midwives to retain registration,
- provide advice to midwives on professional standards and
- promote safe midwifery practice and quality care for women and their families.

There were 13 clauses in the document, which was framed similarly to its British equivalent (NMC 2002; Lawrence & Yearley 2008). Although the Midwives Rules were intended to make midwifery a profession, they actually prevented

Chinese midwifery from being a profession by limiting autonomy. However, the need to prepare and educate midwives for their role had been endorsed by government. The crucial regulatory measures and professional attainments were consolidated during this historical phase. The approved educational institutions at that time were mainly missionary- and hospital-organised.

Rules for midwifery education

Following a midwifery programme extending over at least two years, a midwife was required to pass a national or a provincial examination. The successful registrants could be the students who had successfully completed an approved midwifery programme of education. They should also have been of good character with no criminal record. Alternatively, they could have been practising midwifery for at least three years. The rules mapped a new dimension of the organisation of midwifery in China.

Employment and practice rules

The Midwives Rules of the CMoH prohibited the employment of unqualified practitioners, the mentally ill, those with a criminal record and, especially, women who had had an illegal abortion. People who attended a childbearing woman professionally had to be approved by the CMoH.

They were required to

- be at least 20 years old;
- hold an approved midwifery qualification;
- keep good records;
- make a report monthly to local administrators, giving the name, age, address and parity of women attended and the sex of newborns; and
- keep birth records for at least five years, for examination by the local Health Authority.

There was no clear requirement for renewal of registration in these rules.

Chinese midwives' remuneration may be compared with that of medical staff in order to make sense. According to *Nánjīng* Archives (1003–6–53: 49), in 1946 the average monthly pay for a midwife was 100 to 200 yuan and for a doctor 300 to 320 yuan. Incomes were based on social status rather than workload and achievement.

Shànghǎi *Midwives Rules*

The regulations governing the Registration of Midwives released by the Public Health Bureau of *Shànghǎi* in 1928 were much more elaborate, with 28 articles making it double the size of the CMoH Midwives Rules. It demonstrated all the previously mentioned points (MOGS 1928a, c) and focused on training rules, for example, minimum entry qualifications, length of training, curriculum and entrance examinations.

All midwifery practitioners were required to conform to these regulations. Anyone who had not passed the examination according to these rules was not allowed to practise. The examination of midwives or verification of qualifications was only by a committee nominated by the health authorities of the state or local municipal health bureau composed of distinguished and reputable doctors with biomedical training.

The examination included written, oral and practical parts. Candidates could sit the oral and practical examinations only after they had passed the written examination. The subjects examined were Chinese language, physiology, anatomy, midwifery, hygiene and bacteriology, stressing aseptic technique. An average pass mark of at least 75% in these subjects was required. After passing all the examinations, candidates could be registered to practise.

In *Shànghǎi* any qualified candidate had to be registered with her municipal police station and licenced to practise (MOGS 1928 a, b, c), which also applied to other parts of China. She had to submit her licence for inspection annually. She was required to keep records of the name, age and address of her patients and preserve the data for two years, which is three years shorter than the CMoH requirement. If she encountered problems with a woman's labour, she was required to request the relatives to call a registered medical practitioner or to send the woman to hospital. She should not undertake any operation herself (MOGS 1928a, c).

There were 94 midwives aged between 20 and 46 years old in the first *Shànghǎi* Register in 1928. A minority (37) had obtained their qualification from a midwifery school attached to a hospital, and 11 of them had a telephone number. Their social status appeared to move up to become middle class at that time.

A registered midwife in *Shànghǎi* was forbidden to do anything to induce abortion. Such actions were punishable by law and having her licence cancelled. After attending a birth, she was required to fill in a form of birth report issued by the Municipal Bureau and report the birth within three days. She could obtain from the bureau silver nitrate for prevention of ophthalmia neonatorum and educational literature.

The differences between the CMoH rules and *Shànghǎi* rules demonstrated overtly the different degrees of industrialisation and medicalisation of the areas. Although the rules of *Shànghǎi* stated that they would be in compliance with the CMoH rules, the variations had revealed the different attitudes and approaches in their management in Chinese midwifery. On the whole, the two rulebooks showed China's attempts to catch up with the development of the outside world in a process of reciprocal interaction with missionary colonial medicine, industrialisation and urbanisation.

The regulation of midwifery care is an example of the growth of hierarchies of bureaucrats in maternity care of modern China. It reflects the state's initial recognition of public health as a citizen's basic right. It also confers on the community a degree of protection from the hazards of childbearing and control of the basic standards of maternity care. Ironically, these rules and regulations have been inconsistent. They were not able to be fully operationalised to guide midwives to promote competent practice to benefit mothers and babies.

However, it gradually became generally accepted among the Chinese population that midwifery schools attached to hospitals or universities were teaching in a biomedical model. This did not mean that traditional Chinese midwives had disappeared or they had no clients. On the contrary, they had outnumbered midwives and managed well, simply because people had greater confidence in them as they were familiar, less expensive and more sympathetic to their clients.

Midwifery education

The development of midwifery education in China since the beginning of the 20th century has had to bear the brunt of the wars, political upheavals and drastic economic and technological changes. These developments are discussed here.

Training for traditional birth attendants

Although traditional birth attendants (TBAs) were officially banned from attending births by the *Běiyáng* government of the Republic of China in 1913 (DCPNGC 1913), they were still needed and continued to practise in both rural and urban communities. For the safety of the public, the Nationalist government eventually decided to regulate them and the quality of their service. It issued Management Rules for Traditional Birth Attendants in 1928 (Chinese Ministry of the Interior 1928), treating the TBAs as a group of important carers operating outside the formal maternity care system. They were defined as women attending births without being medically trained or qualified.

The TBA Management Rules of 1928 had 17 clauses, first, to define a TBA and, then, to specify roles, duties, functions and responsibilities. A practising TBA should be aged between 30 and 60 with reasonable health and no infections. She should have attended two months' free training and passed the assessment regarding asepsis, delivery methods, umbilical cord cutting, resuscitation and postnatal care of women and newborns. For illiterate TBAs, the classes would be taught orally. On passing the assessment she could register and obtain a licence to practise. She was not permitted to intervene in the process of labour or perform any operations. Failure to comply with these rules would be punished according to laws, besides having her licence cancelled. She was not allowed the use of any titles other than birth attendant. She sent her records to the local relevant governing body in the first ten days of each month. The records should contain the information of the birthing mother's name, age, home address, parity, newborn's sex and so on and be retained for five years. Her licence under these Rules would expire on 31 December 1931. However, let us not prematurely lament the future for the TBAs. They continued their business as usual because they continued to be needed in their communities, and there were insufficient biomedically trained midwives, nurses and doctors to take their places.

The preceding TBA Rules had to be amended in 1939 by the Ministry of the Interior (1939) under the pressure of a severe shortage of maternity carers. The Rules were extended from 17 to 19 clauses. The age range of a TBA was reduced to between 25 and 50. A registered TBA was asked to fill in a blank form of birth report issued by the local authority and send the same back within the first 10 days of each month. If illiterate, they could ask their client's family to help to fill in the form or, failing that, a police officer, who could not refuse (Article 14). When a licence was lost, a duplicate could be obtained on application and by paying the registration and licence fees and stamp duty as provided under Articles 4 and 5. The licence of a registered TBA issued under these rules could only be valid until 31 February 1941. All these rules were subject to amendment at any time, should any omission be discovered.

The amended rules were more practicable and implementable than those of 1928. The expiry dates of the licence in both of these documents illustrated the government's expediency rather than its principle. The TBAs had obviously been used as a means of extending maternity services to decrease maternal, neonatal and fetal mortality and morbidity before the country had enough well trained, qualified and competent health workers. In principle the state favoured medically trained staff and technological birth. This tendency can be observed in the development of maternity care subsequently.

The first birth attendant school was set up with the approval of the Health Authority of *Běipíng (Běijīng)* in October 1928 by Dr *Yáng Chóngruì* (杨崇瑞), a medical doctor trained by missionaries in Peking Union Medical College (see Chapter 9). The first recruitment of the school was 30 students with an average age of 54 years. In 1928, a total of 360 TBAs were trained in the school according to the Department of Maternity and Child Health of the Ministry of Health of China (MCHDMH 1991: 3; Xia 2007).

The administration of *Běipíng* Birth Attendant School was later transferred to the management team of the Department of Security Headquarters, which was later named the Maternity-Child Affair of *Běipíng* Security Bureau. This transfer suggests a popular perception at that time: that the health of women and children was translated into the security of the larger social order. This required society to police the activities around human reproductive health and the control of child care. This has been criticised by Western feminists as society attempting to control women's profession, body–mind and human reproduction (Annandale 2009: 12–35).

Before its closure in 1932, the school managed to educate 10 intakes and retrained 299 traditional birth attendants (EBFSAMS 1933), but only 96 of them (32.1%) were licenced to practise (for details, see Table 4.1).

One hundred fifty-one midwifery students went through the training. Ninety-six of them registered and obtained their licence to practise in *Běijīng*, and 55 of them had not registered.

At the end of the programme, the school gave each trained birth attendant a basket containing a birth pack and a copy of regulations that would help her apply the sterile procedures and the standards of hygiene she had learnt when attending childbirth. Since then the lay practitioners of '*shōushēng lǎolao*' (收生姥姥) were transformed to *Jiēshēng yuán* (接生员). However, they were still facing

Table 4.1 Birth attendants trained in the Maternity-Child Affair of *Běipíng* Security Bureau

Intake	Licenced	No licence	Deceased/ other	Unqualified	Expelled	Total
1st	15	0	3	11	1	30
2nd	9	1	5	13	2	30
3rd	13	0	6	14	2	35
4th	12	0	3	9	4	28
5th	15	0	4	24	3	46
6th	8	0	2	28	4	42
7th	11	5	2	1	2	21
8th	7	10	3	0	0	20
9th	6	9	1	0	0	16
10th	0	30	1	0	0	31
Total	96	55	30	100	18	299
%	32.1	18.4	10.1	33.4	6	100

Source: EBFSAMS (1933), National Library of China.

difficulties differentiating themselves from medical obstetric practice and laying claim to a variant body of practice-based knowledge of midwifery. The public was suspicious of the quality of their service. In order to secure public confidence, the practices of the newly qualified midwifery graduates were monitored by *Běipíng* Health Authority twice monthly. Their homes were often subjected to random checks by inspectors from the health authority to ensure that they had the delivery basket distributed by the health centre and kept their birth records. These were the basic standards to be expected of them at that time in *Běijīng*.

The trained birth attendants from then on had a duty to ensure that the care they provided was reasonably competent. This meant that they had to be accountable for their actions and their competence in the care they provided. The trained birth attendants and the traditional birth attendants appeared to be battling for survival in terms of safety of newborns and their mothers. By 1936, only 95 out of these 151 trained birth attendants remained in practice and two of those were struck off the register (*Yáng* 2006: 145–6).

Requirements for biomidwifery schools and students

For clinical purposes the Ministry of Education established regulations in April 1936 for midwifery schools and revised them in February 1937 (Chinese Ministry of Education 1937). First, it required that both public and private midwifery schools should be registered with and approved by the Chinese Ministry of Education. Second, students enrolled into a midwifery school were required to already be qualified nurses. Third, teachers were required to already be qualified midwives or teachers and the schools needed to be well equipped. The school was required to be linked to a maternity unit with a delivery room, neonatal room, outpatient department, laboratory, suitable equipment and books. The hospital needed to have at least 25 births each year before being allowed to enrol student midwives, based on the previous year's figures.

According to the 1938 statistics of the Health Experimental Institute of the Central Nationalist Government, there were 32 midwifery schools in the country.

Among them, 3 were state-approved, 15 public and 14 private (HEICNG 1938). Most were closed during the Sino-Japanese War, and the surviving ones were mainly funded by private donations because of a shortage of public funds.

By 1943 the right to create midwives' laws had been transferred from the Health Authority to the central government because of the Sino-Japanese War during World War II. The revised Midwives Laws were released by the central government in September 1943 and consisted of six chapters and 32 items. Apart from the requirements on education, licensing and birth registration, there were regulations regarding the structures of the midwives' associations and confederations. The punishment of those who violated the laws was included. Figure 4.1 is a copy of the signed and stamped instruction by the president of the State Council of the Nationalist Government, which was issued on 11 July 1944.

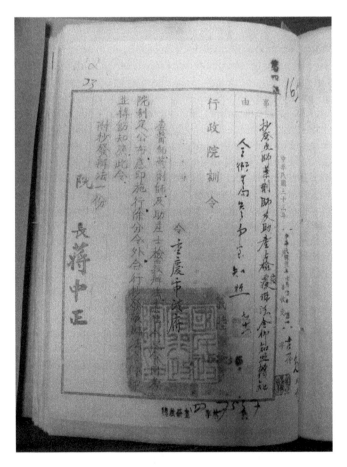

Figure 4.1 The instruction of the State Council

Sources: EBFSAMS (1933), National Library of China.

A state-approved midwifery school

There were only about 500 trained midwives in China in 1929, and most people had to trust in the care of the 200,000 TBAs without formal training (EBFSAMS 1933). Based on what she did previously, Dr *Yáng Chóngruì* (discussed in Chapter 9) managed to persuade the Ministry of Health to approve the first midwifery school attached to a maternity hospital in *Běijīng* in 1929; it was seeking to reach the standard set in the rules. This school became the first of its kind to obtain formal state approval (*Fù* 1986).

At first, this was a two-year programme, following 12 years' schooling approved by the Ministry of Education, but it was extended to three years in 1935. There were no midwifery textbooks available at that time. All teaching materials were compiled by the lecturers, a collection of which became the blueprint for the textbook for provincial midwifery schools (*Fù* 1986). The majority of teachers were from medical schools and some were clinical practitioners. Thus, Chinese midwifery developed through midwifery schools and licensing laws modelled on Western medicine.

As well as training midwives, the School led the development of midwifery and established links with local health organisations. In April 1933 the school established a midwives association (discussed later in this chapter) to strengthen communication and academic exchange.

There were four programmes running in the school up until July 1934:

1) advanced course for midwife teachers;
2) basic midwifery course to train midwives;
3) midwifery research course;
4) nurse-midwife course (EBFSAMS 1933; ECSC 1936).

There were 115 graduates of these courses (Table 4.2).

All students had to obtain one to three months' clinical experience in their subject in the facilitated hospital or Peking Union Medical College Hospital.

Although there were many midwifery graduates, 74.4% maternity care (see Table 4.3) was carried out by birth attendants at that time in *Běijīng*. This table shows the births attended from July, 1932 to June, 1933 in *Běijīng*, illustrating who attended births.

This midwifery school was closed in 1952. Within these 23 years of education, 450 midwifery undergraduates and 136 postgraduates in total had completed their studies there. The postgraduates consisted of 22 refresher course midwives, 50 nurse-midwives, 48 midwife-researchers and 16 midwife-teachers (*Fù* 1986).

Development of this state-approved midwifery school was, with hindsight, a government tactic to impose medical control of midwifery education. State regulation of midwifery practice through licensing laws was also achieved. Having

Table 4.2 Training courses and graduates – *Běijīng* Midwifery School, 1929–1934

Type of Programme	Purpose of training	Length	Intakes	Graduates	Notes
Advanced	Midwife teachers	2 years	5 Intakes	39	Graduates worked in 5 provinces: *Jiāngsū, Shāndōng, Héběi, Shānxī and Shǎnxī*
Midwifery	Midwives	6 months	4 Intakes	32	The training was stopped after these four classes.
Research	Midwives further training	6 months	2 Intakes	13	Graduates returned to where they originally came from.
Nurse-midwife	Hospital midwives	6 months	5 Intakes	31	Graduates returned to where they originally came from.

Sources: EBFSAMS (1933); ECSC (1936)

Table 4.3 The numbers of births attended by school-trained TBAs and midwives and untrained TBAs in *Běijīng*, July 1932–June 1933

Month	7	8	9	10	11	12	1	2	3	4	5	6	Total	%
School-trained TBAs	5	8	4	9	12	21	22	16	18	7	15	13	150	2.7
School-trained midwives	102	100	108	103	97	99	138	115	115	94	90	114	1275	22.9
Untrained TBAs	265	255	293	418	335	352	384	395	408	305	325	406	4141	74.4
Total	372	363	405	530	444	472	544	526	541	406	430	533	5566	100

Source: EBFSAMS (1933); ECSC (1936).

Note: TBA = traditional birth attendant.

confidence in midwives, the Chinese government applied medical power to control midwifery rather than allowing midwifery to develop on its own as an independent profession. The combined forces of medical self-interest and the convenience of state control had created modern Chinese midwifery as an important maternity care profession but subsumed under medicine.

In this context, midwives and obstetricians struggled to establish their own professional boundaries. The state's decisions and actions also contributed to conflicts between midwifery and obstetrics. This was because state policy addressed midwifery as simply one aspect of obstetrics and allowed medical professionals to control midwifery education and its licensing. This historical problem is still waiting to be tackled.

China looked to Europe as a model of how to establish midwifery. In Britain, female reformers campaigned to modernise midwifery and to eradicate traditional midwives or handy-women (Leap & Hunter 1993); this modernisation reduced mortality rates and provided middle class women with a new profession (Towler & Bramall 1986; Donnison 1988; Tew 1998). The Midwives Act of 1902, for England and Wales, created the Central Midwives Board, although initially it was medically dominated. It preserved midwifery as a health care field within the modern health system by privileging trained midwives over traditional midwives (Lawrence & Yearley 2008: 261–82). China wanted to catch up with the development of the world, so it needed to make a foreign midwifery system serve China. It needed to have a structure to regulate, educate and encourage midwives. In China midwifery was treated as an insignificant health issue. The state did not know how many midwives practised in the country, except those worked in the hospitals and in the metropolises.

Nánjīng *Advanced State-approved Midwifery School*

Nánjīng Advanced State-approved Midwifery School (NASAMS; 1936) was set up in 1933 by *Yáng Chóngruì* (discussed in Chapter 9), the same person who had already founded the *Běijīng* State Midwifery School. The period between 1931 and 1945 featured almost unprecedented chaos and disaster in China because Japan invaded Manchuria in September 1931 and created a Japanese puppet state of *Mǎnzhōuguó* in 1932 (Geelan et al. 1974: VIII). This started the 'Anti-Japanese War' (1931–1945), as most Chinese call it. The Sino-Japanese War (1937–1945) eventually broke out on 7 July 1937. Many major cities including *Nánjīng*, *Shànghǎi* and *Běijīng* were occupied in that year by the Japanese. On 28 March 1938 the Japanese established a puppet government in *Nánjīng* (Black 1999: 272). After failing to stop the Japanese, the Chinese government relocated in *Chóngqìng*. This long and disastrous war did not end until 1945.

During the Sino-Janpanese War, the NASMS also withdrew to *Chóngqìng* in the remote south-west. The school was thus under the direct management of the Central Health Authority of the Nationalist government. This is further discussed in Chapter 8. In 1938, because of the serious shortage of midwives, it tried to train birth attendants there and sought placements for its students (Figure 4.2).

After World War II, the NASMS moved back to *Nánjīng* in 1946. Then the civil war between the Nationalist and Chinese communists broke out and intensified. The communist troops took first *Nánjīng*, the Nationalist capital and later Canton, *Chóngqìng* and the entire mainland. The name of the school was changed to the current *Jiāngsū* Medical University for Health Workers.

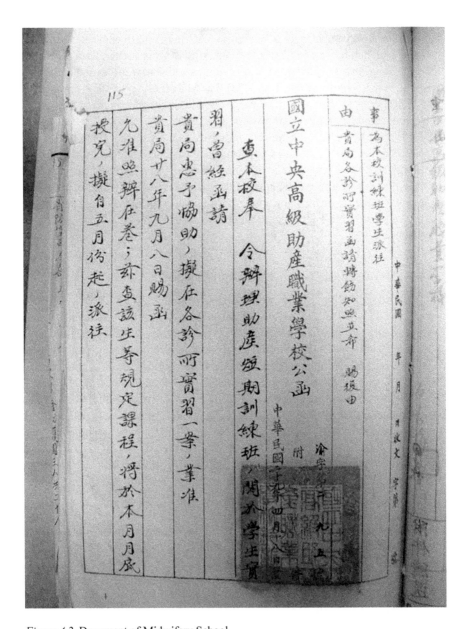

Figure 4.2 Document of Midwifery School

Source: *Chóngqìng* Archives 0066–1–13, p 115, taken by the authors, 2008.

A midwife's certificate and her activities

A certificate was issued by the Examination Committee of the Capital Police Bureau in *Shěnyáng* to Miss *Zhāng*; one of the authors (NFC) has been able to scrutinise this document but permission to reproduce it has been declined. The certificate records that Miss *Zhāng* was born on 22 December 1922, passed all the examinations and was licenced to practise midwifery in July of the eighth *Kāngdé* year, that is 1941 (*Nánjīng* Archives 1003–6–753: 170; see Guide- Chinese emperor's titles and Timeline). There are two basic year markings in Chinese history: the dynastic cycle and the continuous number of year in the way that the BC or BCE is. *Kāngdé* year here is a regnal year starting from 1934, when Manchuria was occupied by Japan and the last *Qīng* emperor was chosen to be *Kāngdé*, emperor of Manchuria, and to have his new palace in *Shěnyáng*. Hence, to change the eighth *Kāngdé* year to CE, eight is added from 1934, making the regnal year 1941.

Miss *Zhāng*'s certificate was confiscated during a search of her home and her belongings by the revolutionary committee in *Shěnyáng* in the 1970s: it was then transferred to the *Nánjīng* Archives after the Cultural Revolution because she was once an independent midwife in *Nánjīng*. The correspondence between these two archivists reveals that her certificate was taken into their custody simply because it was issued by an institution of the puppet government under Japanese occupation. Hence, this certificate was perceived as evidence of betraying the country – not simply for making living. However, her certificate was very lucky to find its way into an archive because the majority of similar documents, deeds and appointment letters issued by the previous governments were retained and then destroyed during the searching and prosecution of the owners at that time. This demonstrates, on one hand, the hardship experienced by Miss *Zhāng* and, on the other, her mobility and the geographic similarity of practice within urban areas in China.

This surviving evidence has shown that the road to a midwife's licence could be a long and rocky one, especially in an occupied territory. First, she had to take an examination when she had completed the theoretical and practical phases of the programme. After passing the examination, she obtained the certificate above which certified her proficiency in midwifery. She was then allowed to register at the local municipal police station and was permitted to practise as a midwife. When the political environment changed, her skills to make a living and serve people became a crime, attracting humiliation and persecution. It may be hard to imagine the circumstances in which she had to study and work as a slave to a foreign power in *Shěnyáng* and *Nánjīng*, Japanese-occupied territories. Additionally, relations between urban birth attendants and licenced midwives certified by an institution held by the Japanese invaders could be very tense and hostile.

Midwifery was one of the most important occupations with greatest opportunity for independence. This could be observed from the two licences issued to *Zhāng Sù-chén* The first was issued by the head of the Department of Health of

Chóngqìng City on 29 May 1942 and the second one by the heads of the Department of Health and the local government in *Sìchuān* Province in April 1944 (see Figure 2.1). Both of her licences met a similar fate as the earlier certificate and ended up in *Guǎngzhōu* Archives, as she was originally from *Kāipíng* County, *Guǎngdōng* Province (*Guǎngzhōu* Archives 5–1–292 and 13–2–56). Ms *Zhāng* was clearly very mobile, either because of the Japanese occupation or her efforts to make a living.

After the Japanese surrender, the five-year civil war between the communists and the Nationalists started. These two wars brutalised the country and brought much destruction, poverty, starvation and devastation to people's lives. The transformation in the urban areas was huge. However, the rural areas remained relatively unchanged. Midwives continued to be active in both urban and rural areas.

Midwifery education since 1949

Since the communist government came to power in 1949, midwifery education in mainland China has imitated that of the Soviet model; this discontinued the higher education and simply kept two to three years' midwifery education in nursing colleges, following nine years of compulsory school education (Cheung et al. 2011c). Hence, we term this kind of education 'secondary' (or intermediate) midwifery education hereafter (see Chapter 6). As to the post-secondary and undergraduate midwifery schools, they were closed. Since then all midwifery schools were either transformed or merged into nursing schools (*Fù* 1986).

A total of 30 midwifery schools and 5,268 midwives in 1949 registered with and licenced by the National Health Administration (Chinese Ministry of Health and Education 1951; Watt 2004: 67), while the mainland population was nearly 600 million in 1953. In order to tackle the serious shortage of midwives, short-term training classes were recommenced for birth attendants from 1951. They were similar to those run in the late 1920s (as discussed earlier in this chapter) but more flexible. Birth attendants could attend a full-time two-week course, or they could attend 50 hours part-time. After the training they were no longer called birth attendants but *jiēshēngyuán* (接生员), who were allowed to practise immediately and then register a year later. The government goal was set for one midwife or *jiēshēngyuán* per 5,000 to 10,000 population. If there were not enough birth attendants to be retrained, the schools would train women activists to be this new kind of birth attendant (*Zhèjiāng* Health Authority 1951).

The emphasis of the course was on antenatal checks, sterilisation of equipment and attending birth. The basic skills learnt included the following:

- recognising signs and symptoms of pregnancy
- calculating the expected delivery date
- washing hands
- cleaning the perineum
- antenatal checks

- using clean scissors and instruments to prevent neonatal tetanus
- umbilical cord care
- breast feeding
- baby bathing
- emergency measures and ways to get help
- keeping brief medical/mortality records

(Chinese Ministry of Health and Education 1951)

Together with other higher education in China, midwifery education was brought to a halt from 1966 to 1971, as it was considered non-essential by authorities during the Cultural Revolution (1966–1977). Thus, existing health services became paralysed. A system of barefoot-doctors was introduced because of the shortage of doctors, medicine and maternity care. The barefoot-doctors were un-/semi-trained staff. Although barefoot-doctors relieved the shortage of medical and maternity care in rural areas, the disruption to the existing care system was detrimental to people's lives (Croll 1985a, 1985b, 1995).

After the calamity of the 10-year Cultural Revolution, the remaining Chinese secondary midwifery education, like other subjects, was resumed in 1979 (discussed in Chapter 10) and improved slowly. Undergraduate nursing education was introduced in 1983 (Smith & Tang 2004) and postgraduate programmes in 1995 (Cheung et al. 2005b), but midwifery still remained secondary and vocational. Less was demanded for care in childbirth, as family-planning policy after 1980 became more aggressive and intrusive, compared with the 1960s. The aim was to restrict the population to 1.2 billion by the turn of the century. In general, a system of incentives and penalties was used to implement the one-child policy and punish those having more than two children.

Midwifery education continues to be a sub-branch in nursing and the content of its education is variable in line with different institutions and their geographic locations. The successful applicants to enter these courses now have to have finished 12 years school education (9 years of compulsory education plus 3 years of high school education). Alternatively, they can enter the course if they have already had a qualification of secondary midwifery education. When the undergraduate students finish their study, they can obtain a BSc degree in nursing with a midwifery orientation. However, this midwifery programme was discontinued in urban areas in 1993 but managed to survive in rural areas in accord with the needs of the society and/or political power, and the existing midwives were transformed into nurses and doulas (discussed in Chapter 5) after 1996.

The educational curricula of midwifery reflected medical dominance, with medical staff involved in programme design and teaching. In the first two years of undergraduate study, courses are shared with medical and nursing students. As a result, many students move into medicine or nursing if they have a choice. The knowledge valued for midwives is simplified medical knowledge rather than matters relating to midwifery care, as midwifery was seen as an adjunct to medicine. After the successful completion of a full-time midwifery programme, the college graduates would be able to get a nursing degree because of the absence of a mid-wifery degree in the education system. However, on the whole, the emphasis of the education has been on nursing/medical skill acquisition of the past practice but not necessarily with analytical and critical thinking skills.

Chinese midwives associations

In this section, three important midwives associations are studied respectively. They are *Běipíng* Midwives Association (BMA), the Midwives Associations of China (MAC) and *Chóngqìng* Midwives Association (CMA). The roles of these associations were to provide advice to midwives on professional standards to protect the interests of the midwives. Although they were not statutory bodies, they could establish some rules and regulations to expel disqualified people from their organisations in order to protect the public interests.

Běipíng *Midwives Association*

As midwifery education developed in China, midwifery graduates scattered all over the country. In order to communicate with each other and to promote Chinese midwifery and its education, the midwives in *Běijīng* set up an association of midwives, worked out the structure and constitution and elected a president, consultant, secretary and treasurer. The president was *Chén Yídí*; vice president, *Huì Huìzhāng*; and consultants, *Yáng Chóngruì* and *Yáng Bǎojùn*. *Běipíng* Midwives Association became established in April 1933.

This Association published a quarterly midwifery journal beginning in June that year and providing a platform for communication among midwives.

National Midwives Association of China

The National Midwives Association of China (NMAC) was established in *Chóngqìng* in 1941, to further standardise midwifery (Figure 4.3a, b). The reason for it to be in *Chóngqìng* was because of the evacuation of the central government there during the Sino-Japanese War. As a result, biomedical midwives gained further ascendancy over traditional practitioners.

The first mission of the Association was illustrated in the application letter in Figure 4.4a, b to *Chóngqìng* Nationalist government to establish a maternity hospital for the poor in *Chóngqìng*.

They raised some funds and submitted their proposals (Figure 4.4a) and the plan (Figure 4.4c) of the hospital to *Chóngqìng* Nationalist government on 12 September 1943 and obtained the permission to build the hospital on 14 October 1943 (Figure 4.4b).

The establishment of the NMAC brought with it ideas of citizenship and responsibility. This maternity hospital opened its doors on 1 September 1944, and the photo in Figure 4.5 was taken during its first anniversary celebrations. The hospital has now become *Chóngqìng* Health Centre for Women and Children, which plays an important role in the life of women and children, and the hospital is well remembered by people there.

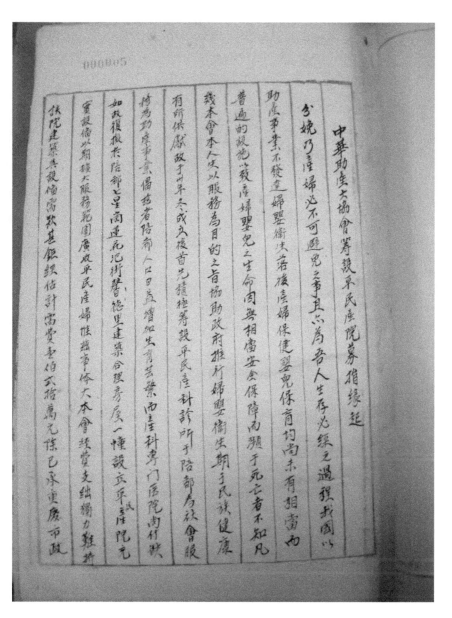

中華助產大協會籌設平民產院募捐緣起

分娩巧產婦必不可避免之事且為吾人生存必經之過程我國以

助產事業不發達婦嬰衛生落後產婦保健嬰兒保育均尚未有相當內

普通的設施致產婦嬰兒之生命固無相當安全保障而頻于死亡者不知凡

幾本會本人夫以服務為目的之旨協助政府推行婦嬰衛生期于民族健康

有所供獻故于卅年冬戌及後首先籌設平民產科診所于陪都后敬會服

特為助產事業備於省陪都人口日益增加生育芸芸產科專門醫院付缺

如我復撤去陪部七星崗建築合擬募屋一幢設立平民產院元

置設備以期擴大服務範圍廣收平民產婦惟茲事體大本會經費支絀欄力難持

欵院建築費設備儲濟欵甚鉅銀頭估計需費壹佰式拾萬元係已承建慶市政

Figure 4.3a Page 1 of the letter written by the honourable chairwomen of the Midwives Association of China

Source: *Chóngqìng* Archives, No: 0060–14–79, p. 5; photograph by authors, 2008.

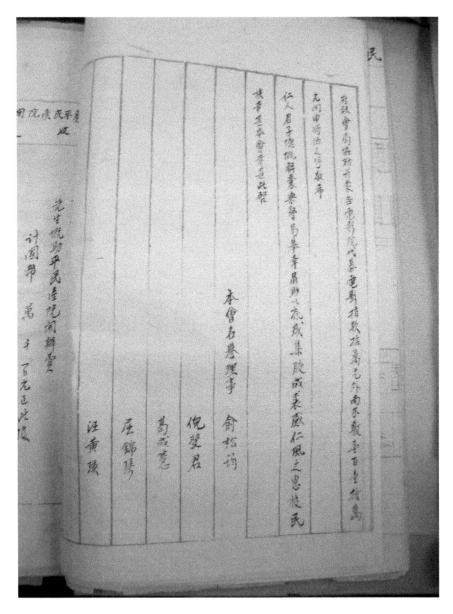

Figure 4.3b Page 2 of the letter written by the honourable chairwomen of the Midwives Association of China

Source: *Chóngqìng* Archives, No: 0060–14–79, p. 6; photograph by authors 2008.

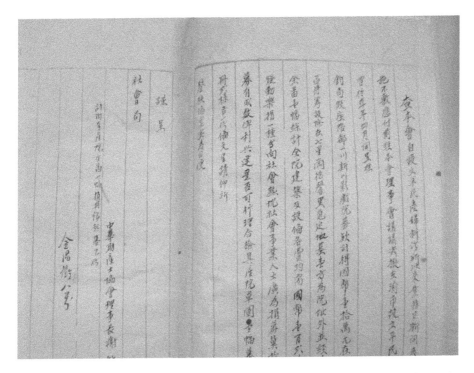

Figure 4.4a The application for a *Chóngqìng* Maternity Hospital for the Poor made by the CMA

Source: *Chóngqìng* Archives 0060–14–79, photograph by authors, 2008.

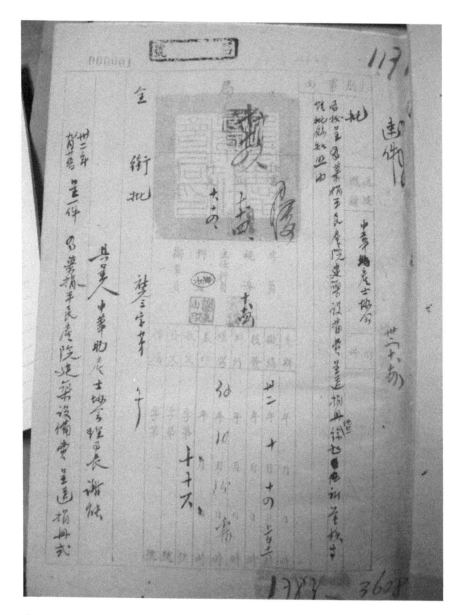

Figure 4.4b The approval forms from the Social Welfare Bureau

Source: *Chóngqìng* Archives 0060–14–79, p 117; photograph by authors, 2008.

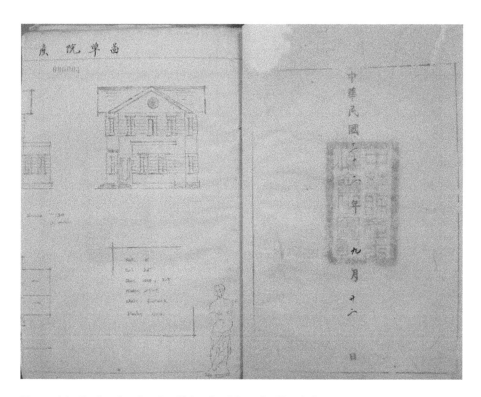

Figure 4.4c Design drawing for *Chóngqìng* Maternity Hospital

Source: *Chóngqìng* Archives 0060–14–79, p. 4; photographs by authors, 2008.

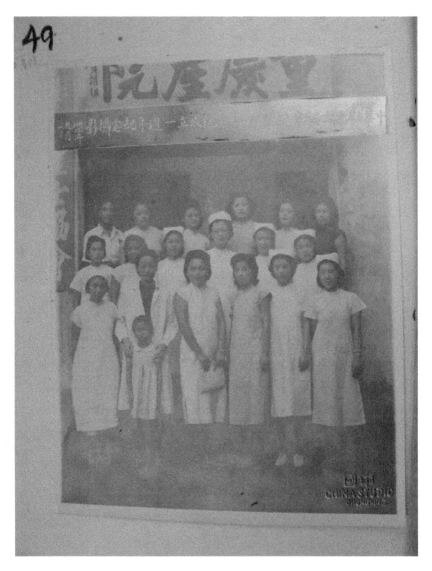

Figure 4.5 The photo was taken on the first anniversary of *Chóngqìng* Maternity Hospital for the Poor on 1 September 1945

Source: *Chóngqìng* Archives 0170–6–1, p. 49, photograph by authors 2008.

Chóngqìng *Midwives Association*

The CMA was a local midwifery organisation initiated by eight midwives in 1946. They were *Xiè Yàomíng, Yú Yúnzhēn, Zhèng Huàguāng, Liáng Guīfàng, Tán Bǎoqín, Yáng Huìyīng, Wáng Jiāxián* and *Yáng Mínghéng*. The inauguration of the CMA was held on 13 June 1946, and 34 people attended, including 29 members; two officials from the *Chóngqìng* government, one from the Department of Social Welfare and the other, from the Health Authority; and a secretary. The meeting passed a 29-item constitution for the CMA, which was composed of more than 200 midwives. The purposes of the association were to promote communication among midwives and assist the government to eradicate untrained midwifery practice and illegal abortion. Figure 4.6a is the record of this inauguration and signed by the chairwoman of this CMA and Figure 4.6b is the list of names and brief CV of each of the founders of the *Chóngqìng* Midwives Association.

No material was found in regard to the continuing activities of the preceding three midwives associations after 1949. Since then all midwives associations have had to be merged into the Chinese Nursing Association (CNA) and become a CNA's sub-branch: Obstetric Nursing Committee (Li & Guo 2009b: 31).

Development of Chinese midwifery

Developments in Chinese midwifery and maternity care must be interpreted against a background of national crisis. The educated elite in China between 1928 and 1949 worshipped pure science, technology and trade in much the same ways as 19th-century Westerners did. Maternity health care in *Běijīng* started a training course for traditional midwives in 1928 and exercised strict control over the midwives. As a result, the biomedical midwifery schools managed to stay and grow slowly in the urban areas throughout the country.

Overpopulation became a subject of public debate in the mid-1950s, and the practice of human population control was adopted as official policy. However, with the Great Leap Forward in 1958 there was a reversal of official policy; a large population and the largest possible labour force were regarded as economic assets rather than liabilities. The great majority of the Chinese population remained rural and agricultural. Midwives played a full role at this time both in the urban and rural areas (discussed in Chapter 10).

The health policy-makers of the new government overlooked the advances in industry and science that were taking place in Western Europe and North America as ideologically incorrect. They kept on seeing themselves as living in the Middle Kingdom, which was superior to all others. This surreal attitude towards the outside world was to bring China much grief, as well as serious problems in midwifery, since the mid-20th century.

Since there are no specific legal or governmental rules or associations specifically for midwives, the title and jobs of midwives have not been protected by law since the communist party assumed power. The previous pre-1949 regulations

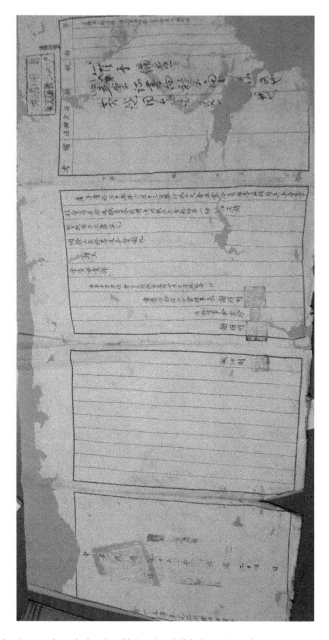

Figure 4.6a A record made by the *Chóngqìng* Midwives Association

Source: *Chóngqìng* Archives 0051–2–543, p. 2; photograph by the authors, 2008.

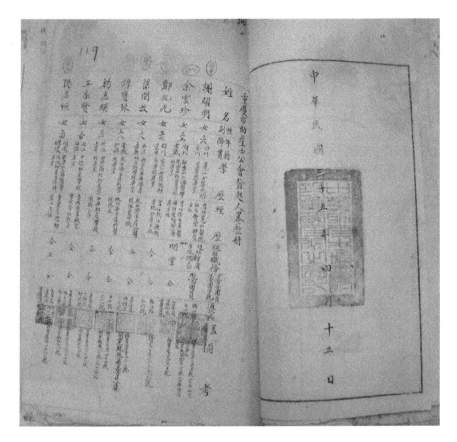

Figure 4.6b The name list of the founders of the *Chóngqìng* Midwives Association

Source: *Chóngqìng* Archives 0066–1–12, p. 119; photograph by the authors, 2008.

and associations were abolished by the new government, and there has been no replacement since. Worst of all, there has been no higher education or continuing professional education for midwives. However, life continues and, at the time of writing, families are expanding. Commonly nowadays, obstetricians, nurses and doulas assume the role of midwife in Chinese hospitals, and midwives are fighting a losing battle in the maternity services.

Unfortunately, under the influence of the obstetric model of North America, Chinese midwifery and the preparatory education were thought non-essential and discontinued in 1993. Midwives were replaced by doulas by 1996 (Cheung et al. 2005b, 2009a). The demise of midwifery education has been complete because few midwifery, but more medical students, have been trained in China since 1972; among policy-makers and the public, obstetricians were considered better-trained and safer practitioners than midwives. Therefore, health policy required obstetricians to take over midwives' role in normal birth to meet the target of 100% hospitalisation of childbirth (CMoH, UNICEF, SC 2003), although statistical evidence indicates that mortality for hospital births was no lower than that of GP units or planned home births (Tew 1998: 343–4).

The changes in Chinese midwifery care have had contradictory and double-edged effects. In China, midwifery has been denigrated by health authorities (CMoH, UNICEF, SC 2003), despite midwifery's global development. In China, there were 30,000 population per midwife (CMoH 1999), compared with 1,500 per UK midwife (Peate & Hamilton 2008). Simultaneously, traditional birth attendants are four times more plentiful than midwives in China. It is difficult to describe these dynamic developments in Chinese midwifery in simple, relatively static words. Many maternity services provided by doctors have become highly sought after, though costs have increased and there are dangers of excessive intervention. Provision of essential information and the right to give birth naturally are often unavailable to women, especially the poor. It has been shown earlier that governmental policies are important for the functioning of midwifery and maternal/child health services. A study of this topic is overdue and would yield important conclusions.

A case study: new biomedical delivery in Bādōng County, Húběi Province in 1986

In order to know how many women gave birth using the new biomedical approach, Wu and Zhang's study (1987; Figure 2.1) was undertaken in December 1986. A random sample of six districts, including 18 villages, 154 village groups and 401 new mothers in Bādōng County, Húběi Province was used. The respondents had to be mothers and their relatives who had had babies in 1985.

The researchers found that 42 out of 126 villages or towns in this county had no midwife or birth attendant at all. A majority (53.62%) of women (215/401) in the sample had a 'new' biomedical birth and among them, seven (1.75%) gave birth in hospital. The remainder were attended by traditional birth attendants. Because birth attendants could not reach a pay settlement, a 32 of 34 birth attendants stated that they worked on voluntary basis. There was no local government funding provided to support the care of women and children.

The discontinuation of midwifery

Xinhua News Agency (1980) reported that midwifery training had recommenced in Běijīng in 1980 after a 15-year break; this happened because at that time only 27 of 130 staff in Běijīng (population 9.04 million then) were trained midwives who were working in the 16 urban and district hospitals there. The hospitals in suburban and rural areas had hardly any midwives and the majority of women were looked after either by medical staff or birth attendants. The quality of the maternity service was greatly affected by the shortage of midwives, and neonatal mortality was increased from 7.35% in 1978 to 10.8% in 1979. Table 4.4 shows

Table 4.4 Maternal and child mortality rates per 1,000 births in the survey areas in China

	Total		Urban		Rural	
	2004	*2005*	*2004*	*2005*	*2004*	*2005*
Maternal mortality (/100,000)	48.3	47.7	26.1	25.0	63.0	53.8
Neonatal mortality (%)	15.4	13.2	8.4	7.5	17.3	14.7
Infant mortality (%)	21.5	19.0	10.1	9.1	24.6	21.6
Mortality, under 5-years-old (%)	25.0	22.5	12.0	10.7	28.5	25.7

Source: CMoH (2008a).

the mortality rates of neonates, infant and children under five in the other areas in China. Forty female students were then enrolled in *Běijīng* Second School of Health Study. The midwifery programme lasted for two and a half years. It was certainly good news to have a small midwifery programme restarted in *Běijīng*.

The interruption in midwifery education and practices may be explained in terms of wars, political campaigns, heavy industry, modern science and technology. Looking back at history, these seem to be the essentials and priorities in the process of building and modernising nation states. The national well-being, such as health care, including maternity care, came far behind these priorities. Very often, a nation state was built against other nation-states. It must appear stronger before it could resolve its weaknesses. This is a political paradox. Inherited from a medieval empire, with a very loose social infrastructure, the modern Chinese state faced an enormous task to resolve its internal weakness while finding a foothold in the world of nations. In this aspect, China was not dissimilar to other nations, even though the tasks they were facing were all different. The modern British state did not oversee its midwifery education until 1902 (Donnison 1988: 161; Tew 1990: 54). The US had its first nurse-midwifery school in 1939 when, because of the Second World War in Europe, the few American centres offering midwifery care were no longer able to send midwives to be trained in Britain (FNU 2018). At the same time, as we have pointed out earlier, the rise of modern medical science and technology, even in times of economic prosperity, diminished the already low professional status of midwifery in many modern nations. By the end of 19th century and well into 20th century, the North American and other English-speaking Commonwealth countries relied more on obstetric doctors than on midwives for childbirth among the rich. Midwifery education declined in these countries. As a result, the poorer and the isolated communities were often served by inadequately trained midwives, who further damaged midwives' professional reputations in these countries (Tew 1990: 53). Such a situation was not very different from what happened in China at the end of the 20th century.

Many medical staff had not mastered the skills and arts of normal birth (Huang 2000) because their performance was assessed on their expertise in instrumental deliveries. The dominant medical culture and the increasing incomes of families and health workers led to a rapid rise in caesarean rates from the average of 18.1% in 1991 to 34.7% in 2004 in urban settings (Li & Shi 2004). This was further confirmed by the WHO global survey on maternal and perinatal health from 2004 to 2008 (Lumbiganon et al. 2010; Souza et al. 2010). A total of 373 institutions from 24 countries in Africa, Americas and Asia were recruited and 286,565 births were analysed. The overall caesarean rate was 25.7%, but China's caesarean rate researched 46.2%, the highest of all. Caesarean without medical indication in China was performed for 11.6% of all births. A total of 63% of all caesareans without medical indication were performed in Chinese institutions ($n = 1,689/2,685$). There is now a great demand for the return of midwifery services (Cheung et al. 2005a, 2009a; Cheung 2009).

Discussion

This chapter has explored the highs and lows of Chinese midwifery and the diverse experiences of Chinese midwives from 1928 to 1996. Midwifery was moved from domestic or private settings to the public sphere. The evidence presented here bears direct witness to the events, people, and processes of the moment. Although rules, schools and associations for midwives were established in 1928 and 1941, respectively, the Chinese midwife's professional development did not progress despite the great efforts made by midwives, midwives associations and the state.

The precise causes of the decline of Chinese midwifery remain obscure; it does, though, show a close link with the absence of a state policy for midwifery, a national higher education for midwives or a national midwives association since 1949, in addition to the implementation of the one-child policy. Further research is clearly needed to identify the precise social status of midwives within their communities of different regions and to reveal why Chinese midwifery took a 'downturn' particularly after 1949. However, the demise of Chinese midwifery has illuminated the importance of the profession in many perspectives. Notable is the absence of, first, university-level education; second, professional regulations; and, third, a national association protecting the public from unsafe midwifery and improving childbirth and the health of childbearing women. These perspectives are unfortunately steered by an ideology of supremacy of obstetric technology and have led to a shocking caesarean epidemic spreading inexorably across the country. As a result, the control of technology is emphasised rather than quality of care and development of midwifery.

The decline of Chinese midwifery also highlights poor understanding of physiological childbearing and the inadequacy of national health policy and state legislation. Wars and revolutions in 20th-century China only aggravated such inadequacy. Imported midwifery practices and educational systems did not meet the needs and demand of physiological childbirth. Leaving Chinese maternity services to the working of the free market imposes more interventions and costs and is not likely to offer a better solution. These issues are further addressed in the next chapter.

5   Recent midwifery developments

Three new developments since 1997 have followed the nadir of Chinese midwifery and have fundamentally changed the experiences of women and midwives there: Chinese 'doulas' (Cheung et al. 2005b), a midwife-led normal birth unit (MNBU; Cheung et al. 2009a, b, 2011a, b; Mander & Cheung 2006; Mander et al. 2009), and the establishment of the first midwifery research unit (MRU) in China. The first two are paradoxical in regard to the advancement of midwifery. In order to understand and further the development of midwifery, the midwife research unit (MRU) was developed, and it stimulated further midwifery studies in China.

The Chinese 'doulas'

The fashionable practice of 'doulas' attracted the authors' attention in 2004 in an international collaborative study of Chinese caesarean decision-making. It was followed by more in-depth interviews until this phenomenon was explained with 27 health workers and 22 women. The questions related to who the doulas are, what roles they have and why they are needed (Cheung et al. 2005b).

The quest for knowledge about Chinese doulas was nothing more than 'common sense', which changes across cultures. The term *doulas*, but not their practice, was introduced into China in 1996, and its meaning was extended to the practice of the privately hired 'doula-nurses/midwives' for financial reasons. This service was welcomed by more affluent families because they were the only supportive birthing companions allowed in the labour delivery room (LDR). Probably most important, this practice redeployed LDR nurses/midwives and retired midwives trained before 1993 because managers had stopped employing midwives and transformed them either into doctors in rural or nurses in urban institutions. Doula-nurse/midwives provided one-to-one care to labouring women and conducted the birth if currently employed. Their role ended two hours after the completion of the third stage. The rationale for them was the need for midwives and the need for re-evaluation and re-integration of Chinese midwifery into the health care system.

The Western doula and her duties

An extensive literature search has demonstrated that *doula* was originally a Greek term meaning a 'woman slave, a woman servant, a laywoman or a maid' (Mander 2001: 113–33; Doulas Australia 2004; Doula UK 2017; DONA International 2017). It has been amended to denote a mother's helper in the home after the birth and then a birth companion, losing any derogatory meanings. Despite all these changes, the term *doula* is not used in childbearing in Greece.

Women have helped other women give birth since the dawn of time. However, organised doula services have only appeared recently in the US, Canada, Australia and other countries. One of the largest organisations, Doulas of North America (DONA), was founded in 1992 (Nunn 2005), currently having trained and certified more than 5,000 doulas worldwide (DONA International 2017).

In North America, there are two types of doula – for birth and postpartum. The birth doula supports a labouring woman and her partner. As a non-professional health practitioner, she can offer a range of comfort measures during labour, such as massage, aromatherapy, reassurance and coping techniques. The postpartum doula is a supportive adviser, helping with newborn care, caring for any older children, family adjustment, food shopping, meal preparation, school runs and light housework. Her role is similar to the Dutch 'maternity home care assistant' (van Teijlingen 1990) and '*yuèsǎo*' in China (Cheung et al. 2006b). Therefore, US doulas are perceived as becoming the first line of assistance for birthing families (Jackson 2005). As well as reminding the mother of her birth plan and empowering her during labour to be her own best advocate, they also remind care providers that they are dealing with a human being with human needs.

However, Jackson (2005) reports that a few certified doulas in the US 'deliver' babies as well, but they differ from midwives. Unlike midwives, they are not trained to deliver the baby. They function like traditional birth attendants (TBAs) in China in the past, apart from their functions as women's advocates. US doulas are trained and certified by their organisations, while TBAs learned their trade mainly through personal experience.

The 'doula' in the UK is similar to those in the US in that she is a professional labour supporter and/or postnatal helper (Doula UK 2017). She differs in that she is not legally permitted to plan to deliver babies, and a midwife or medical practitioner must supervise her and attend the birth. Doulas in the UK are normally mothers themselves, trained by their own organisation and supported by various health professionals.

The doula has been welcomed by some childbearing women in the US as helpful in meeting their needs for non-medical support. She may contribute to the solution to what has become known as the caesarean 'epidemic' (Mander & Cheung 2006). For these reasons, in China the introduction of the doula has also been welcomed. It is not certain whether this welcome in the US is justified, based partly on the Dublin experience (Hodnett et al. 2004). Women in Dublin who had continuous, one-to-one support, albeit often by unqualified and inexperienced personnel, during labour were less likely to have a caesarean. The introduction of doulas in China appears to be more complicated according to the literature and Cheung et al.'s study (2005b).

The Chinese doula and her duties

The 'doula' in China (Sun 2005; Zhai 2005) means a privately hired LDR nurse or midwife providing one-to-one care during labour. Less is known, though, about how a Chinese doula performs these functions. There are no antenatal or postnatal doulas in China. In terms of duties, a Chinese *yuèsăo* (Cheung et al. 2005a) does a similar job to a postnatal doula in North America, and the Dutch maternity home care assistants (van Teijlingen 1990).

To make sense of the practice of the Chinese 'doula' we have to pull together the cross-cultural knowledge of Chinese midwifery and the Western doula. The loan term *doula* to refer to LDR nurses and midwives was adopted by the Chinese to indicate modernisation of midwifery in terms of humanity and individuality (Zhai 2005); this is because foreign-sounding interventions are thought to indicate novelty and attract more buyers of their services. Therefore, the doula has become a symbol of the globalisation of maternity care there and has replaced the services provided by LDR nurses and midwives.

Doula in China takes its meaning from its purpose but not from its Western functions and structures. It has a close relationship with Chinese midwifery under local conditions, local needs and local cultural perceptions.

The appellation of the practice was adopted from North American countries, mainly the US, which was often seen as innovative by many Chinese intellectuals, who had run out of inspiration after many stagnant years. But in three aspects – the economic, the political and the cultural – the Chinese had developed the doula with Chinese characteristics who differs from the North American doula.

In North America, doulas were initially organised as a way to provide one-to-one, humane birthing care locally and to encourage normal birth and discourage obstetric intervention and hospitalisation. The Chinese, though, saw this care in economic terms. Although doulas resembled traditional Chinese midwives, their one-to-one services had become a commodity for a market price when a woman was in established labour. This practice, on one hand, offered a route for Chinese midwives to re-enter their LDR territory, because of the state's attempt to replace them with obstetricians and nurses since 1993 and to promote 100% medical deliveries in 2003 (CMoH et al. 2003). On the other hand, it has also split the midwives' role into doulas and obstetric nurses. As a result, this further aggravates the demise of midwifery and loss of the social and professional identity of midwives in China.

Politically, the presence of doulas is affecting the role of the midwives, who in China have been reduced to doulas, that is, a mere technical role, rather than the holistic role promoted as the ideal in the UK. This 'technocratic' role (Davis-Floyd et al. 2009: 456–60) is reminiscent of the LDR nurses so familiar in the US. As a result, the midwifery role is under threat by effectively being split into its two component parts.

Culturally, the Chinese 'doula' stands at the crossroads of several streams of cultural influence. One is the obstetrical orientation (see Chapter 10); second is a Chinese response to the introduction of doulas in the West; third is the needs of labouring women; and, finally, there is the need for the deployment of redundant midwives.

To sum up, the 'doula' in China has been transformed into an ethnocentric and culture-bound term. It means LDR nurses/midwives offering, for the market price, one-to-one support during labour. Although the number of doulas providing services was small in the hospitals, the publicity they received was overwhelming. Hence, 'doula-midwife' is used here instead of doula in order to avoid any confusion with the Western meaning.

Who are the doula-midwives?

According to the head of a maternity hospital involved in our fieldwork in 2004, the concept of doulas was first initiated in Shanghai in 1996. They were recruited from retired LDR nurses and midwives employed in hospitals, as the hospital staff reported being too busy to cope with their daily routines. These doulas were aged between 55 and 65, had some experience and were happy to take on this task. Their role, to be with women during labour, compelled them to assist women to strive for a vaginal birth, but unfortunately, they were not allowed to deliver the baby because of their age. Their pro-vaginal birth approach led to conflict with the existing LDR staff because they wished to get their job done quickly so that they could have a bit more time for themselves. In order to avoid such conflicts between the LDR staff and the doulas, the hospital administration then decided to deploy LDR staff to be doulas as well.

From then on, Chinese doulas consisted of both the currently employed and the retired LDR nurses by training and midwives trained before 1993. All of them call themselves 'midwives', but none of them is a registered midwife. They are nurses by employment and registration, simply because there has been no national register for midwives in China since 2001 (CMoH 2001, 2012). The confusion over their identity has prevented them from making a positive connection between their position and the midwife role; this has sometimes prompted them to complete the birth quickly and has resulted in an instrumental delivery or caesarean operation.

The age of the retired doula-midwives was considered the reason for them not being allowed to deliver babies. There were no courses at the outset designed specifically for them; neither were there courses designed for LDR nurses and midwives to update their knowledge and skills. Only recently, courses for training doulas have been mushrooming, as offering these courses has become a viable form of income generation. This indicates a different local conception of midwives and their roles. It not only reflects but also reinforces the Chinese health authority's desire to structure its service comprehensively at the lowest cost. It is this distinctive response to the doula phenomenon that attracted our attention.

In addition, the above phenomenon posits a hierarchical ordering in terms of the relationship between a Chinese doula-midwife and an LDR staff member. This provides a basis for our analysis: a structural contrast between Chinese doulas and Western doulas.

What does a Chinese doula-midwife do?

According to our respondents, if the family could afford and were willing to pay for doula services (as the birth fees did not include one-to-one care), an on-call doula-midwife would be called from her home when the woman is in established labour to attend her and the birth. They would stay with and look after the woman, encouraging her to take food and drinks, massaging and supporting her.

A doula in China differs from a Western doula by possessing a much broader and deeper understanding of the technical processes and concerns, because all of them have been LDR trained nurses or other health workers. If she was a current LDR nurse/midwife, rather than a retired LDR midwife, she would also deliver the baby when labour progresses smoothly. Since the involvement of current LDR staff, the retirement-aged doulas are gradually disappearing from doula care, especially when the demand for their services has declined.

No woman interviewed for the study (Cheung et al. 2005b, 2011a, b) reported that any supportive birth companion was allowed to accompany her during labour. This was because the presence of family and others was considered, by the LDR staff, inconvenient to their management of the labour. A doula-midwife was the only person allowed to be in the birthing room to support vaginal birth; this was because the labour room was usually shared by many labouring mothers and was considered to be too crowded to accommodate any other birth companions.

Chinese doula-midwives left the woman two hours after childbirth. There were no postpartum doulas in China. The postnatal care would be taken over by the women's families, '*yuèsǎo*', '*yuèzǐ bǎmǔ*' (Cheung et al. 2005a) or a domestic nurse for the first month (Cheung 1997; Cheung et al. 2005b).

The doula-midwife's practice emphases the relations between biological needs and cultural life. It was in a way women-centred. The 'doula' care distinguishes itself from standard hospital services. Therefore, the service of doula-midwives was regarded as enhancing the woman's status and the quality of the care she received (Cheung et al. 2005b). This transformation by the doula raises some questions. Did the doula services *cause* the fragmentation of Chinese midwifery? What was doula care in essence? How should we see the role of the midwives? Why did the delivery fee not include the one-to-one compassionate care as standard?

Training

The introduction of the doula into China has become a route by which LDR midwives may return to practice, which has also, however, split their role. According to a health worker interviewed, the hospital managers organised their own pool of doula-midwives and provided training if required. However, there was no specific doula-midwife training programme reported for LDR and retired midwives in 2004; since then, various training courses have mushroomed throughout the country. As China does not have a national midwifery education system and a special training designed for midwives, it was for the aspiring doula-midwives to update their knowledge and practice through self-directed learning, attending nursing degree courses and/or talks organised by the hospital.

Confusion still exists about the role of a midwife and the clinical and social needs for her services. This is reflected in the fact of the absence of national registration and employment system for midwives in China. Maternity service providers consist largely of doula-nurses and LDR nurses who have an additional three months' on-the-job training (Pang 2010) to prepare them for their role. They were considered midwives simply because they were working in the labour rooms and doing part of a midwife's job; an obstetrician doing a midwife's job, however, remained a doctor. The presence of 'doula' services becomes an issue for concern for the midwifery profession. The problem of appropriate training for midwives can only be resolved through national recognition, regulation and the re-establishment of proper midwifery education.

The issues of quality or safety of practice did not appear to be a problem to the LDR staff in the study and the doula phenomenon was regarded by them as merely a matter of a name or naming. What mattered was to get the job done. Nevertheless, it appears that these LDR staff are not in the best position to question a development such as the role of a midwife, the arrival of the doula, or other forms of medicalisation. It may be argued that education in the role of a midwife, as identified by the International Confederation of Midwives, is very much needed to make Chinese maternity care more effective and woman-oriented.

Pay

The pay scales of health workers in China, as set by the government, have been very low nationally. Similar to other civil servants, they have traditionally been given performance bonus and additional allowances by their hospitals for housing, travel and other benefits to supplement their basic pay. These supplementary incomes can comprise over 90% of their monthly salary. This has been one of the main causes of corruption to push both the public and private sectors to look for other possible sources of income generation; such sources include increasing unnecessary clinical examinations, pharmaceutical treatments and operative interventions to generate supplementary income.

The pay for the retired doula-midwives was about 7 to 8 Yuan/hour (70–80 pence/hour) for day duty and 10 Yuan/hour (£1/hour) for night duty. As to the hospital-employed doula-midwives, they would earn a bonus to their monthly salaries, similar to the medical house officers, which amounted to 6,000 to 10,000 yuan monthly. Their salary and bonus would vary in different hospitals, different regions and according to the time spent. The charges to the birthing women varied between 300 and 100,000 yuan, in addition to the birth fees for using the doula-midwife service.

What does doula mean?

The name *doula* means LDR nurses and midwives who are one-to-one birth companions. The practice of doulas in China is the response of the maternity services to pressure from consumers and from the development of Western midwifery practice. The service providers responded by the adoption of the term of *doula* only but not its practice. However, there are certain boundaries that cannot be crossed. The doula must be a trained nurse and/or midwife or doctor. Therefore, the findings mentioned earlier should be interpreted with caution. They provide only a snapshot of the situation in China at one point in time and may not represent the changing situation. They demonstrate how Chinese midwifery has developed over a difficult time and how they have responded to the 'caesarean epidemic'. In spite of these limitations, it has relevance to other communities and can inform the meaning of Chinese doula in areas where change is slower.

In this discussion we, the authors, focus on two issues: the differences between the doulas in China and Western countries and the rationales for the transformation of Chinese doulas.

Differences between Chinese and Western doulas

In Cheung et al's study (2005b) four distinctive differences were identified in relation to the Western doulas.

First, Chinese people were indifferent to the original meaning and practice of doulas. 'Doula', in the West, is a lay labour supporter and/or postnatal helper, whereas in China, her function is more like a TBA, *yuèsăo* or home helper. The doula in China was not associated with the TBA but was transformed into a doula-midwife. Such Chinese indifference indicates concern for utility and novelty seeking for profit.

Second, the exotic term *doula* was borrowed in a manner of 'enlightened' and 'modernised' self-interest in China. This self-interest implies a reciprocal relationship to ensure a mutual accommodation between the service providers and the service users. This term was only accepted on condition that it served these purposes, especially on the side of the service providers.

This became obvious through the absence of other supportive birthing companions during the labour. The doula-midwife was usually the only person allowed to support women having a normal birth. This practice is different from that of the West. For example, in the UK the constant presence of a birth companion of the woman's choice is perceived to be one of the most effective forms of supportive care in childbirth introduced in the last few decades (MIDIRS 1996, 2005). These support people may be the woman's partner, family members, friends or trained laypeople such as a doula; they provide emotional and informational support, physical comfort and advocacy. In China in spite of the clear benefit of continuous labour support, only a doula-midwife was recognised as a supportive person in labour. This clearly indicates that woman-centred care is secondary to the convenience of the service providers.

Third, the doula was introduced by the system as a cheap option. This was because no training was required for existing labour ward staff to be doulas, as their routine job was to care for labouring women.

Finally, the service of a doula has become a unique selling point (USP) there, because it satisfies three distinct aims. It provides, first, a midwife with an opportunity to practise her midwifery skills; second, to focus her care on a one-to-one basis; and, third, to obtain some extra income to offset her ever-rising living costs. This increased self-interest and an increased ethnocentric definition are their defence against increased pressure from the outside development of midwifery.

These identified differences earlier led the authors to search for the causes of these changes.

Rationales for the transformation of 'doula-midwives'

The service of a doula in the West is similar to that of the existing Chinese TBA. However, the services of a Chinese doula have never been associated with a TBA at all but, rather, have been assumed by a LDR nurse/midwife. This orientation has five interpretations.

First, on the surface, it is the inevitable outcome of taking something foreign without fully understanding the original meaning. However, this would be too simple to take as a misunderstanding. The term *doula* has provided a convenient means of demonstrating becoming 'modernised' while yet remaining 'Chinese'. This symbolic function will be further discussed later.

Second, it is the persistent desire on the part of service providers to structure maternity services cost-effectively by every conceivable means – including the manipulation of the meaning and practice of the doula. Managers have been anxious to promote a progressive and modernised image both at home and abroad. The indifference of the health authority to the understanding of the Western doula illustrated their utilitarian attitude and their profit motivation.

The selective indifference to current Western meanings, practices and the nature of women led to the development of the present doula-midwifery services. To this end, the economic incentive was important for its introduction. Both the service-providers and the service users were seeking to promote their individual interests at the expense of the collective interests of Chinese midwifery. Such behaviours ultimately led to the creation of doula services that are profitable to the institution and their staff, though low value relative to midwifery as a profession and blatantly high cost to consumers.

Third, doulas were introduced into Chinese hospitals to promote a one-to-one maternity service. Its practice in China was different in the mechanism the health authority chose to emphasise. The exploitation of the term *doula* permits the development of the transformation of doulas, which signals a utilitarian thinking in pursuing status gains in addition to the economic gains mentioned previously. This strategy is a political and economic solution to a problem of low-standard maternity services. The intent is apparently not a measure to achieve the modernisation of Chinese midwifery but to exploit the resources of the transactional meanings of 'doula' and its local re-interpretation in the light of symbolic meanings.

Fourth, the value of the term's use was to transmit a message that the hospital care was comparable to Western services. This symbolic intent was not only related at micro-exchange level (Turner 1991: 333–51) to the interests of women. More important, it related at a macro level a symbol to the service providers' advantage in the process of social change initiated by the technological modernisation and the promotion of maternity services.

In China, the doula is a symbolic presentation indicating modernisation for midwifery's supportive care during birth. This symbolic approach to foreign ideas and practices is deeply embedded in the Chinese consciousness. This indicates that the development of doula services is a result of local imaginations and its practices are inseparable from its cultural context. Such an approach may have led to the argument for the fundamental illogicality of science. This naivety not only reflects that consumers' access to suitable information is insufficient at all levels of society (Cheung et al. 2005b) but also reinforces certain features of traditional, stereotypical characteristics, such as conformity and acceptance without question.

Culturally, the doula becomes a symbolic resource that is certainly regarded by the health authorities as 'the unique selling point' for their services. The continuous, one-to-one care provided by doula-midwives during labour has been perceived as an innovation in childbirth. It illustrates the woman's need for a midwife and the status needs of midwives and their system.

Last but not least, having the full attention and assistance of a doula-midwife was not surprisingly perceived by Chinese women as a positive experience. It would immeasurably increase the self-esteem of a woman as a woman and a mother if her family could afford it.

China has its traditions, communities and human resources to provide women with birthing companionship and supportive care. Labouring women have been helped by female relatives and/or friends since time immemorial. But unfortunately, they are not allowed into the labour ward, because the hospital does not treat this custom as a system. The service of doula-midwives was created as a commodity and a symbol. These practical concepts of purpose, rationale and utility constitute the rudiments of a basic theory of a Chinese doula service.

Based on the findings, we argue that the concept of 'doula' is only meaningful in terms of the community to which the women belong.

The introduction of the transformed doula illustrates and reinforces the need for midwives, the need for a re-evaluation and re-integration of Chinese midwifery as a system and a need for a cultural awareness and understanding of the influence of globalisation. The supportive care provided by a midwife and a birth companion is based on the recognition of its kind. The health authorities should acknowledge it and assess the needs of service users.

A midwife-led normal birth unit

The second important development in the recent period was the establishment of the first alongside MNBU in China (Cheung et al. 2009a, b, 2011a, b; Cheung 2015). The development was intertwined with politics, culture, diversity of practices and economic incentives. Iatrogenically high caesarean rates alarmed us and led to a funded exploratory study on caesarean decision-making (CDM) in China. The main CDM findings were the demise of midwifery, over-reliance on nurses, obstetricians and technologies and the absence of evidence-based research information for informed choices (Cheung et al. 2005a, b, 2006a, b; Mander & Cheung 2006).

Informed by the above findings, the first MNBU was designed. After two years of preparation, the unit was eventually established in *Hángzhōu* in 2008 with 'two-to-one' intrapartum supportive care (midwife, birth companion and woman), face-to-face, virtual (communications and consultations) and tele-midwifery care (e.g. video classes, video monitoring and inquiries). The vaginal birth rate in the unit was 87.6% in the first six months and has remained between 90% and 94.8% ever since. The episiotomy rates have been steadily falling from 77.8% to 43.2%. Midwives there have taken pride from their 24/7 service as both safe and positive experiences (Cheung 2009; Cheung et al. 2009a, 2011a, b, c; Mander et al. 2009). They have also derived a sense of self-worth, self-esteem, and have learned to differentiate themselves from other health care providers.

This was confirmed by a story told by one of the midwives:

> I have been a midwife for over thirty years. When I just started this job, I had the instinct to provide the compassionate care for women, but my effort was soon dismissed by the existing busy maternity system. I'm glad that I have eventually learned through working in this Midwife-led unit. It helps me to understand and confirm eventually what midwifery is and how a midwife should work. I'm also glad to be able to understand, finally, after these years, at nearly the end of my career, that the safe supportive care during childbirth is essential for a midwife; and it is the essence of midwifery.

Demand for MNBU services is increasing and voiced all over the country. The following story of a second-time mother expressed this view:

> I had a lovely normal birth in this unit. It is great to have my husband and the midwife with me throughout the labour. That was very reassuring. They always offered me a cup of drinks, a relaxing massage and made a little chat. When my birth was getting difficult, the midwife stayed very cool and kept on explaining, encouraging and reassuring me and my husband. The rapport developed during the antenatal care and the labour allowed me to feel confident and to make through the labour.
>
> The birth I had previously in my home-town helps me appreciate the care I had in this unit. I've never seen this kind of good service before. It is excellent! I hope this kind of wonderful service can be available everywhere in the country

The midwife-led care (MLC) success is because of research leadership, midwives' commitment, participation, international collaboration and the continuum of care. More important, it empowers women to shape their experience according to their own definitions and it depends on the interactions of women, their families and communities with midwives.

This is ground-breaking for this hospital. The MLC outcomes came to the attention of local politicians three years later. The city council has mandated and funded centrally that all midwives in the city must work in the unit for three months, to be exposed to the philosophies, skills and techniques used there so that they can be taken back to the other hospitals (Downe 2011).The unit was able to accept 34 staff from the other institutions across the country for training in 2011.

This model constructs the understanding of the link between midwifery and normality. It illustrates how the power of the kindness and compassion of midwifery care can change the system and promote normal birth (Pan & Cheung 2011). It also shows a concise understanding of China's political, social, human and economic systems that are what makes China tick.

Unfortunately, the policy for appropriate staff ratios has been lagging behind the development. Based on the earlier experience and supported by the first newly established MRU (as discussed later in this chapter), midwives took active parts in the four years (2010–2014) international COST Action IS0907 (COST 2010); and hosting the Normal Labour and Birth, the 7th International Research Conference in *Hángzhōu*, China in 2012. Through these interactions and exchanges, the first national Midwifery Expert Committee (MEC) was established in 2013, the committee and its midwives are pledging their engagement in calling for the government's political and legal commitment to address its neglect and responsibility. A way forward is being sought.

A midwifery research unit

The preceding two developments led to the birth of the first MRU in China in 2008 at the School of Nursing, *Hángzhōu* Normal University. The major goals of the MRU were to launch studies to improve the understanding and the development of midwifery education and practice. The years that followed saw three tremendous engagements: collaboration with international institutions in midwifery research, advocacy for normal labour and birth, and the International Confederation of Midwives (ICM) Gap Analysis Workshop (GAW). The last but not the least added greatly to the understanding, development and prestige of Chinese midwifery.

Research

The MRU actively engaged in the study, development and evaluation of the MNBU (Cheung 2009; Cheung et al. 2011a, b, ; Pan & Cheung 2011; Renfrew et al. 2014) and has led to important changes. It stimulated and assisted the formation of *Zhèjiāng* Midwives Association and becoming a member of the ICM; this was in spite of conditions causing all midwives to transfer their professional identity to that of nursing and medicine. It organised a cross – institutional Chinese research team to take part in and co-hosted by the University of Central Lancashire, UK, the 7th Normal Labour and Birth Conference in 2012 in *Hángzhōu*, China (see Figure 5.1).

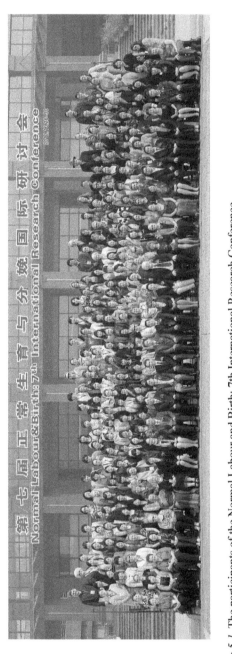

Figure 5.1 The participants of the Normal Labour and Birth: 7th International Research Conference

Source: Provided by the organisers of the conference.

The key participants of the Conference undertook an important workshop on the state of Chinese midwifery in China in 2012. It was agreed, after heated debates, to carry out an ICM GAW in the subsequent years in order to strengthen midwifery profession and improve its services in China (as discussed later).

The MRU also participated actively in the successful COST Action IS0907 (2009–2014): 'Childbirth Cultures, Concerns and Consequences: Creating a Dynamic Framework for Optimal Maternity Care'. MRU focused on the experience of internal migrants in China to challenge inequality in maternity care there (Cheung & Pan 2012). It reached its height and made a keynote presentation on its understandings and findings of 'Bridging Culture and Practice – The Cultural Approach to Midwifery' at the ICM 30th Triennial Congress: Midwives: Improving Women's Health Globally in Prague, Czech Republic, in 2014. This participation in the Congress involved a delegation from mainland China for the first time.

'Normal birth'

The MRU has argued that 'normal birth' is the essence and the theory of midwifery; it is a process of understanding of one's own body. Though *normal birth* is a simple term, it is far more complicated in theory and in practice. It concerns women's health in relation to the problems of medicine and medical technology. A theory of 'normal birth' can be developed in terms of family life, antenatal, intra-natal, postnatal and neonatal care. 'Normal birth' can be understood from the perspectives of both the sociology and the anthropology of health.

The controversy over the definition of the term *normal birth* has implied its complexity as the issues of the doula and MNBU discussed earlier. To define what 'normal birth' means we have to learn and to understand what health, illness and culture are. The question of the controversy comes out of the problems of social and cultural changes. As we have changed our lifestyles in the progress of industrialisation and socialisation, we have changed our ideas about what is normal and abnormal. If we think that changes are normal in our cosmos, then normality should be viewed as a dynamic concept. We may think about a multi-definitional approach contextualised in space and time. We may find we will talk about 'to improve what is normal' rather than 'to keep what is normal', and the essence of 'normal birth' in our human societies is the idea of 'care'. What care we can provide will lead to what we think is a normal and healthy birth. The idea of 'care' is to improve the physiological process and will certainly eliminate all unnecessary interventions. If the idea of 'normal birth' conjures up all theoretical questions about birth, the content of 'care' tests these questions in practice.

Normal birth as proposed by the MRU is not a rejection of science but a scientific process of understanding of birthing health in complex systems. The MRU prompts Chinese midwives to participate in international research, such as a four-year project on the 'Childbirth Cultures, Concerns, and Consequences' of the European Cooperation in the field of Scientific and Technical Research in 2009 (Downe 2009). 'Normality' is closely related to 'salutogenesis' (Antonovsky

1979, 1987) and 'complexity' (Downe 2008, 2009). The findings of the MRU inspire Chinese professionals to explore midwifery further.

ICM membership

In order to address the issue of midwifery development in China and understand fellow midwives in the other part of the world, 100 midwives established the *Zhèjiāng* Midwives Association (浙江省助产学组) (an affiliate of *Zhèjiāng* Nurses Association). They joined the ICM in 2008 to become one of the 121 autonomous associations from countries throughout the world and the first ICM member from mainland China.

ICM GAW

It was against this background that the concept note was worked out (see Further Reading and Notes – The International Confederation of Midwives Gap Analysis Workshop in China) and a two-day the ICM GAW was proposed in 2013 to look into the issues of education, regulation and association of the development of midwifery in China. Against the odds (see Chapter 11), the workshop eventually obtained approval and support from the ICM and the National Health and Family Planning Commission (NHFPC), and now the National Health Commission (NHC) in 2018; and funding from the ICM and *Shíjiāzhuāng* Maternal and Children's Hospital.

The three ICM gap-analysis assessment tools and four core documents were first translated into Chinese and then sent to 16 stakeholders in April–May 2013. Eleven completed forms were returned (return rate (RR): 68.75%), analysed and interpreted.

Forty leaders in these three areas including the GAW respondents were invited to attend the workshop in *Shíjiāzhuāng* on 26–27 March 2014, but over 120 leaders and experts arrived. They included stakeholders, NHFPC policy-makers, senior representatives from the ICM, the Chinese Maternal and Child Health Association, Chinese Nursing Association, the Society of Perinatal Medicine, Chinese Medical Association, Women's Association, higher educational institutions, the United Nations Population Fund (UNFPA) and non-governmental organisations in China.

The workshop aimed at reaching an in-depth understanding and consensus by discussing the findings of the survey in China in relation to their expertise and responsibilities. The workshop focused on studying the *ICM Definition of a Midwife*, the *ICM Essential Competencies for Basic Midwifery* and the global standards for the 'Three Pillars' (UNFPA et al. 2011): midwifery education, regulation and association (ERA).

The findings of the three tools were analysed and compared in the fashion they were designed for. The tools are straightforward, even though the interpretation of the answers is less so. The analyses and assessments of the developments in these three areas are reflected and illustrated in a matrix to reveal the situation, understanding and future actions are in China. The gaps identified are listed in Further

Reading and Notes – Gaps identified by the assessment of the ICM Gap Analysis Workshop to facilitate comparison.

The gaps identified are mainly the absence of definition, higher education, national registration and regulations for midwives at policy level; the lack of a national association and a professional ladder at clinical level and a lack of partnership and interactions at an individual level. The GAW concluded with a joint 'Call to Action' (see Further Reading and Notes – Call to Action) for the development of midwifery in the coming years.

It sets out the vision, mission, commitments and actions for midwifery development as a long-term strategy to improve the health and overall well-being of women, newborns and families.

The first government response to the call to action was the approval of a trial development of a BSc degree programme in eight key universities in China, even though the appointed institutions were still unsure how to move forward. Then it was followed by the establishment of a 'national midwives association' the under the newly established Midwifery Expert Committee of the Chinese Maternal and Child Health Association in 2015. It seems that midwives in China are preparing to work with the experts and governmental, regional, and national levels to develop programmes and policies to address these gaps. This co-operation will elevate the availability, acceptability, affordability and quality of maternity care provided by midwives.

Discussion: learning from the past: challenges and progress

This chapter has presented three major developments in Chinese midwifery since 1997. The first concerns the interrelationship of the concept and practices of doulas in China, which is not a sound practice but simply letting the commercial product known as 'doulas' be affordable to consumers.

The second development, of the MNBU, challenges the obstetric-orientated system in China. It questions how kindness, compassion and respect matter in maternity care and how they work to generate their effects (Cheung 2015). The recent national and international research collaborations, including the ICM Gap Analysis, the COST Action IS0907 and the Normal Labour and Birth, the 7th International Research Conference led by the MRU in *Hángzhōu*, have already encouraged midwifery practice there. These have initiated a favourable shift of the system from one that was about safety only to one that is about both safety and positive experiences.

Last but not the least, the MRU is actively engaged in research in childbirth, midwifery education and practice (Renfrew et al. 2014). Through the ICM Gap Analysis Workshop, the status of midwives was given due recognition. An understanding of genuine humanity in midwifery care and culturally specific practices was achieved through the workshop, with due recognition of the fundamental rights of women and newborns.

The concept of 'normal birth' adopted by the MRU and the call to action after the ICM Gap-Analysis Workshop would further women's sense of coherence [an orientation put forward by Aaron Antonovsky (1979: 160–81, 1987: 15–32) through one's dynamic confidence to search for the origins of health rather than the causes of disease], returning midwifery to its rightful place in education and the care of healthy childbearing women. The unit's continuing research in future would definitely add to the understanding of midwifery and 'normal birth' in China and in the international context, facilitating contrast and comparison.

Part II
Current situation and issues

'Professionalisation', 'modernisation' and 'marginalisation' are issues which need to be understood for midwifery to become an important part of health care. These are concepts which cause concern and are discussed in other industrial societies in different social and cultural contexts. In the midwifery service with China's particular social and cultural background, the presence of and social aspirations in these issues have their own characteristics. However, with globalisation, different social and cultural values, ideologies, theories and practices of science and technology infiltrate more into economic, social and cultural life; thus, the current state and development of midwifery are no longer isolated phenomena which, perhaps, they may never have been. We need to see development from the perspective of social and cultural exchange and impact, and we will reveal differences and similarities of midwifery practice between different social and cultural backgrounds. The current state of midwifery and related issues cannot be separated from historical development; therefore, the understanding of history and tradition is integrated throughout the three parts of this book.

A more rational shape of maternity care with modern goals for China, the complexity, theory and issues of midwives' 'marginalisation' and overcoming it, and professional co-operation is discussed in depth in this part.

6 Midwifery and its professionalisation

This chapter examines the relations between the profession and professionalisation (Freidson 1986), the legitimacy of Chinese midwifery, the practice, power, and rivalries over claims to knowledge and skills and other issues. The concepts of profession and professionalisation are often contested and used by practitioners to gain prestige, and by organisations as a tactic to regulate the members of an occupational group. These require constant transformation of midwives' embodied knowledge, which must be sustained by individuals and their organisations. Such grounding requires detailed analysis of how organisations work and how Chinese midwives using their organisations are differentiated by their social position and their application of knowledge.

The biomedical model of Chinese midwifery is a result of modernisation, a product of social transformation and a development of scientific human knowledge. Midwives' concepts are socially constructed and vary according to different groups in pursuing their occupational strategies and maintaining their different cultural contexts (Mann 1983). This chapter explores how Chinese midwives work on their professionalisation; we illuminate tactics and strategies that occupational and professional organisations might use to initiate changes in the profession.

According to Freidson (1970a, b), a profession is founded on the self-interest of members seeking power or control, which affects how this group organises their jobs and controls their resources. The exclusion of disqualified members would promote the peer groups to obtain statutory approval and gain professional competence and accountability, supposedly, in the public interest. These devices serve to discipline and, thus, control and regulate the members' conduct. This self-disciplinary control of the members brings us to the issues of autonomy over working conditions; also associated are changes in the balance of power which a profession requires and issues of the relationship between political and economic interests, responsibility to society, legal obligation, and cultural identity. There are many ways in which these elements can be dealt with, such as integrity, objectivity, professional competence (ICM 2010), confidentiality and accountability (ICM 2014). As to the obligations of a profession, we should not overlook the implicit or explicit value of the group's occupational loyalty or cohesiveness. This may imply the existence of structures or an institution for the public good.

Professionalisation (Mander 2001: 3–4) is a process closely related to the development of knowledge with an emphasis on 'training' to become a professional (Carr-Saunders & Wilson 1933). An institution strives for professional status and to promote the interests and standards of its individual members, the profession and the public. This discussion of the tactics of professionalisation may motivate the professional group members to regulate themselves to facilitate and induce changes in Chinese midwifery.

This chapter illuminates arguments relating to searching for professional power, to generate public support and improve the social status of midwives. This will secure a better understanding of midwifery and facilitate their location of professional autonomy over their working conditions and practices.

Traditional midwives: practitioners or professionals?

The term 'professional' has been used by Chinese historians (Lee 1999; Leung 2000), in the gender and historical debates, to refer to traditional Chinese medicine-men, healers and birth attendants from 618 CE to 1909 CE (see Timeline). The choice of this word, in our view, has more to do with convenience rather than with careful consideration of the variables in their organisation of care.

The concepts of professions are socially constructed and vary from one country to another to explain how human work is organised. Unlike countries in Europe and North America (Radcliffe 1967; Ehrenreich 1976; Donnison 1988; Marland 1993), China did not have any documented competition between male-dominated (man-)midwives and female midwives until recent decades. Only recorded was the struggle between traditional midwives and modern biomedically trained midwives (Huang 2000; Cheung 2009), all of whom were female. The former needs to be neither approved nor regulated while the latter needs to be both. The differences between them relate to who would have control over the birth process. Technical interventions emerge as a predominant modern midwives/obstetricians' unique selling point (USP) in China, to the extent that the misuse of instruments has been and remains common enough among them.

In a modern sense, the ideology of professionalism entails altruism, accountability, social norms and idealism (ICM 2010, 2014; AAT 2014). In other words, the functionalist perspective on professions embraces professional attitudes, a body of systematic and generalised knowledge and embodied skills, professional behaviours, and a concern for the interests of the community, rather than solely self-interest. However, these conceptions have been challenged, notably by George Bernard Shaw and by many sociologists who have been less willing to accept the professional's own idealised representations of themselves (Shaw 1946; Freidson 1970a, b, 1986). Shaw maintained that professions are 'a conspiracy against the laity' (Shaw 1946). He made little attempt to understand the actions of a profession which sought to hide medical errors and lapses in the standards of care.

Professionals have been seeking the monopoly rights within the division of labour and using instruments to maintain their sphere of influence or independence. Taking these meanings into consideration, we cannot help asking how traditional Chinese medicine-men, healers and birth attendants from *Táng* to *Qīng* dynasties (618–1911 CE; see Timeline) could have all these insights into and awareness of the modern concept of professionalism (van Teijlingen 2001: 115).

In traditional Chinese midwifery, China had never been short of self- or privately trained midwives and medicine-men, for example, *Sūn Sī-miǎo* (581–682 CE), *Wáng Tāo* (670–755 CE) and so on. Although they were good at, and compassionate about their jobs (Fu et al. 1982; Liang 1983; Lee 1996; Leung 2000), they were not, in any sense, equivalent in the modern sense of professionals controlled by a code of ethics, established and maintained by a special association and having learned skills by the training required to be qualified persons.

Clearly traditional midwives did not possess the organisational structure and the ethos of modern professional midwives. No obvious historical evidence has suggested a sociological definition for professionalism in Chinese midwifery. However, there were Chinese terms to refer to people of all walks of life around 220 CE, namely, *sānjiào-jiǔliǔ* （三姑六婆）, *sānshíliù héng* （三十六行）, and later *sāngū liùpó* （三教九流; see Guide – Chinese glossary). These so far have only suggested that people were categorised by what they actually did, but not necessarily by how they were organised. They could simply be individuals who carried out similar trades or jobs.

Since medieval times, there have been *hánghuì* (or *hong*, 'the guilds') in urban China, but they were not regulated by the imperial government, and they often became secret societies while undertaking their business or trades. In times of political or economic crisis, these societies became the instigators of revolts against the emperors. We have not been able to learn whether such guilds ever existed in ancient Chinese health provision, including midwifery. We may also ask whether in imperial China there was any rationale to appeal to midwives for them to be organised or 'professionalised' in terms they might have thought of or, at least, in terms of some sort of association. Nevertheless, before and in early modern times, midwives were overseen by medicine-men in China, while in Europe midwives were controlled by men of the church or local authorities. Hierarchies, manifestly related to gender hierarchies, would arise among these different health providers, though we have not found any rationale for these hierarchies, or whether any rationale was needed in the then prevailing Chinese social order. But still, midwives occupied a relatively well-respected place, albeit lower, in society, given the importance of giving birth and being born in society and the experience required of midwives. The respect and importance of such a job could have formed the base for an aspiration for high standards, which, among others, characterises the modern industrial notion of a 'profession'. What was disconcerting was the unequal value assigned to medicine and maternity care. The relationship between midwives and medicine-men would never be that of professions unless these inequitable values were overcome. This has still not happened, long after China has established an industrial social order equivalent to that of modern European societies.

The European idea of 'professions' in the modern industrial era is known in Chinese as something like 'special employments' or 'special business or career'.

There was no awareness of the growth of professionalism until the development of scientific knowledge and technique during the early 20th century.

History: the legitimacy of Chinese midwifery

Legitimacy, from a historical point of view, means the social acceptance and recognition of a practice.

In ancient China if people showed that they understood the dualism of *yīnyáng*, they were legitimated to be healers. For example, the first medical book *Huángdì-nèijìng* (*Wáng* 762) was based on this traditional *yīnyáng* theory. This book is still being recognised as a viable systematic Chinese medical textbook.

Yīnyáng theory was not accessible to all. Many medicine-men were leisured, relying on the gentry's patronage and not having to work for money or practise full-time. These amateurs legitimised their study and practice by caring for patients. They had, for centuries, questioned the principles of *yīnyáng*, which were then incorporated into traditional Chinese medicine. The principles of *yīnyáng* were not controlled by an ethical code but were learned in training. The knowledge and skills of the amateur practitioners were not self-conscious in terms of wider social function and organisation. This knowledge and these skills had not been credited by laws and customs with professional autonomy. The practitioners did not usually publish what they claimed to be useful.

As mentioned already, many medicine-men pursued medicine as a hobby or charitable activity which contributed to their success and popularity, for example, *Biǎn Què* and *Sūn Sī-miǎo* (Wu 2000). They had other interests and means of making a living (Lee 1996). This group of medical amateurs coexisted with commercial practitioners who lived on fees and sales of their herbal medicines (Furth 1987).

Traditional midwives were often illiterate, resulting in few historical documents surviving (Lee 2008: 126–7). Like medicine-men, they looked after their fellow women as a compassionate or charitable activity, which contributed to their success and popularity. Some might have had other interests and ways of making a living (Lee 1996; Chapter 9). Their legitimacy for practising midwifery rested on their duty to care for women. These amateurs also coexisted with commercial practitioners earning fees (Furth 1987).

Before the 19th century, people could claim to be healers or midwives once they had obtained the confidence of clients. This was usually achieved via the head of the household, a male, as China was, and still is, a patriarchal society, especially with regard to health care and childbirth (Furth 1987). The legitimacy of midwifery knowledge was believed to be further enhanced by cumulative life experience; shamanistic prayers, inherited or tested; and secret practices that had been passed down through many generations (Furth 1987). These forms of legitimacy gradually gave way to codes of conduct of midwifery practice set up by the regulatory bodies of the state after 1928 in midwifery, although they did not disappear completely. The changes in the legitimacy of Chinese midwifery have reflected the social changes in response to global cultural diffusion and indicate a dimension of professionalisation of Chinese midwifery.

This discussion of the legitimacy of medical and midwifery knowledge can also be found in the research by Lee (1999, 2008) and Leung (2000). The legitimacy was treated as if it was a typical feature only in a specific period that was under discussion. However, looking at history in this way we may lose sight of the continuity of historical development of Chinese midwifery, reinforcing a call for midwifery professionalisation.

Chinese midwives' roles and identity

The regulations including the Midwives Rules issued in 1928 by the Central Government (CMoH 1928) played a key role in developing the first register and the professional role of Chinese midwives. There were 94 midwives aged 20 to 46 on the First Register of Midwives in *Shànghǎi* (MOGS 1928b). A total of 36 of them were trained by missionary hospital schools in China; one in Japan, and the remainder did not state the place of training. The home telephone numbers given by 11 midwives probably reveal their middle-class origins and social status. The statutory laws governing their registration opened a new era of regulation and control of midwifery practice through educational reform and introducing changes to the profession to produce a new generation of midwifery practitioners: reformed traditional midwives, *jiēshēngyuán* and biomedically trained midwives.

Despite gender prejudice and historical bias, Chinese midwifery has, nevertheless, emerged with the development of western medicine, as a profession which claimed the field and gradually increased its body of knowledge, specialist routines and ideas and its midwives associations (see Chapter 4). This process of having its own schools (see Chapter 4), own associations and developing its own unique knowledge, accountability, control of training and recruitment, autonomy and monopoly of practice and expertise constitute professionalisation (Freidson 1970a, b, 1986; ICM 2011a, b). It has drawn on more education for women and more knowledge of western science and standardised midwifery through educational and licensing requirements.

The 1928 Midwives Rules (see Further Reading and Notes – Midwifery policies in China) delineated a basic understanding of Chinese midwifery professionalisation and were reviewed in 1929 and again in 1943 (Chinese Nationalist Government 1943). Thereafter, many young women benefited from the opportunity to earn a living by working as a midwife (see the examples in Chapters 9 and 10). School-trained midwives gradually replaced untrained or apprentice-trained midwives in hospital settings. Technological professionalisation of Chinese midwifery became necessary for its survival as a profession, although it has not been very successful (Wajcman 1993: 69; ICM 2014). After 1952, midwifery higher education was abandoned, and midwives' own associations (see Chapter 4) were also disappeared by merging into those of nursing. Post-nursing and secondary midwifery education in nursing schools (see Chapters 4 and 10) became the only educational channel for midwives, and it gradually disappeared, especially since the implementation of the policy of total hospitalisation of childbirth (Table 3.2; CMoH et al. 2003).

Feminists' claims to control reproduction and restore women's control of their own bodies became better known in the 1970s (Firestone 1971; Oakley 1980; O'Brien 1981). This movement passed unnoticed in Chinese maternity services. Currently, the total hospitalisation of childbirth still dominates: China has neither a national register for midwives nor a statutory body to safeguard the interests of the public nor a professional organisation for midwives. Chinese midwifery has thus been marginalised gradually; it reached its nadir by 1996, after the introduction of the North American 'doula', which had led to great confusion about the role and identity of midwives (discussed in Chapter 5; Cheung et al. 2005b).

Occupational groups have often used their technological knowledge to make claims of specialisation or professionalism. Technology is, therefore, a key to power between and within professions and service providers and service users relationships (Wajcman 1993: 69–80). But the crucial question is what technology can entail in Chinese midwifery. Midwifery was thought by health authorities to have a direct correlation with malpractice and a relatively high maternal mortality (People's Daily 2002). Midwives are considered by the ICM to be most appropriate for keeping childbirth normal, enhancing the reproductive health of women and the health of their newborns and families (ICM 2018: 32). We can see that in China midwifery has not been thought of as a technical job because it does not involve much technical knowledge. In this instance, midwifery skills in counselling and knowledge of humans and society have been disregarded. Why have Chinese midwives failed to obtain the recognition of their skills in their country? So far, this question has been answered only partly, and we will continue to explore it further.

Gender and childbirth

Human societies have historically divided themselves into two social categories: male and female. This binary biological division of humanity constitutes a sociological debate between nature and culture or sex and gender (Helman 2000: 108–14). Nature is conceptualised as rooted in biology and as fixed, while culture is seen as being changeable and dependent on environment and social contexts.

Sex means the anatomical differences, for example, chromosomal, reproductive, hormonal and other physiological characteristics. *Gender* involves the social or cultural and psychological aspects linked to males and females through particular social contexts (Marsh et al. 1996: 269–316). Feminists have argued that gender differences are a part of a social structure which has placed women at a disadvantage or subordinate to the male, in terms of power and status (Wajcman 1993; Marsh et al. 1996).

Gender bias views women as stereotypically more 'natural' than men. They are said to have a natural instinct to nurture, making them more suitable for family-oriented activities. Male biology is said to make men more aggressive and competitive and therefore more suitable to provide economic support for the family. This biological division of labour positions midwives in the Chinese cosmological *yīn* system, while obstetricians are equated with the male world, or *yáng system*. The metaphors used for female systems are often negative and demeaning by contrast to the male system, suggesting power and positive qualities. How medical science views women's and men's bodies has consequences, both in the rate and the kind of technological intervention. This is exemplified in the different treatments of reproductive disorders in women and men, and in childbirth. With the exception of the limited input of urology, there is no medical speciality equivalent to gynaecology for males. Some feminists argue that this could be interpreted as medical refusal to see the male reproductive system as potentially defective (Wajcman 1993: 68). As well as the long-standing medical interest, childbirth is becoming a focus of increasing public interest in the 21st century.

In childbirth, obstetric technology has undoubtedly been beneficial to some women in terms of life-saving treatments, pain relief and augmentation of prolonged labour. However, it presumes male medical control over women. It is increasingly evident that women are far from being individually in control of their own childbirth and are surrounded by rules, customs, prescriptions and sanctions.

Chinese midwives, like their clients, are becoming regarded as less experienced in attending normal childbirth than male doctors, who possess technical knowledge and skills that midwives are perceived not to have. Thus, the relationship between obstetricians and midwives is characterised by their gender and status.

Midwifery education

To promote the midwifery profession, education, a regulatory framework and the development of a professional organisation are fundamentally important (UNFPA et al. 2011, 2014). Education is, the first of all, key to being professional. The biggest challenges facing midwifery education in China is midwives' marginalised status, through the apprenticeship and vocational training systems.

The survey of the International Confederation of Midwives (ICM) Gap Analysis Workshop (GAW) in China (see Chapter 5) in 2014 reveals that university-level education in midwifery is still not on the agenda. There is no officially recognised definition of a midwife or a university degree or employment for her. 'Midwives' become the carers who only offer women essential birthing care in labour rooms. Their public identity can be obstetric nurses, doulas or obstetricians. They actually are graduates with a certified or accredited two to four years of nursing or midwifery training, though these programmes vary in content and duration and may not include midwifery skills beyond medical and/or nursing training. They are nurses or doctors by employment and education and midwives by apprenticeship. They become midwives after three months' labour ward experience according to Ruyan Pang (2010), vice-chairwoman of the China Maternal and Child Health Care Association. The standards and the content of their education and practice are inconsistent with the ICM requirements (2010, 2011a, b).

The respondents of the ICM GAW survey also reported according to what they understood of basic midwifery training/education, started in 1908 in private schools (see Chapter 4). In 1954, midwifery schools were merged into nursing schools (see Chapter 4). Midwifery education restarted in 1980 (see Chapter 4) and vocational education in 2000. *Chóngqìng* developed an in-service midwives' training course in 2010 to provide post-nursing continuing education and training. The course runs for three months, twice a year, and has been successfully run seven times. This confirms midwifery education in China was either at secondary midwifery education, nursing education or as in-service training.

In 2001 the Ministry of Education in mainland China published the first national policy for midwifery secondary education (see Chapter 4): 'Midwifery mentoring programmed in the secondary vocational schools education'. In our study of the government of health and educational policies we discovered that for some unknown reason, in the same year, the Ministry of Health abolished 'midwives' as a category in the national health statistics. This means all the midwives counted before, since then either counted as obstetric nurses in urban areas or obstetricians in rural and remote areas. The communication and collaboration between these two Ministries seem to have got lost somewhere.

None of the respondents in the ICM GAW survey was sure how many schools offered midwifery education in the country and whether they were publicly or privately funded, because of the absence of statistics. One respondent reported that there were more than 200 schools offering midwifery courses. The authors' studies, however, show that in 2010, there were 301 nursing schools (57 at provincial level and 244 at regional/city level) providing secondary level midwifery training/ courses after 9 years or 12 years compulsory education (Pang 2010). In 2012, we were told by one of our personal contacts in *Běijīng* that these were increased to 349 secondary level and 101 college level. However, a bachelor's degree programme in midwifery was being planned in Beijing funded by the United Nations Children's Fund (UNICEF) and Chinese Maternal and Child Health Association (CMaCHA) in 2012. Figure 6.1 shows the research group, some postgraduates, experts and administrators invited to a meeting to discuss the curriculum they had developed.

In response to the joint 'Call to Action' issued by the representatives of 42 organisations and institutions attending the ICM GAW (see Chapter 5; Further Reading and Notes – The International Confederation of Midwives Gap Analysis Workshop in China), the government appointed eight key universities in 2015 to offer a midwifery undergraduate course (BSc in midwifery) with immediate effect. They are *Běijīng* University, Peking Union Medical College, *Fùdàn* University, *Tānjīn* Medical University (TMU), Southern Medical University (SMU), *Sìchuān* University, *Zhèjiāng* Chinese Medical University and *Xīān Jiāotōng* University. Since then none of them have offered BSc in midwifery apart from two (TMU and SMU) which already had an ongoing BSc in nursing undergraduate course with midwifery orientation since 2006. The successful students of this course have been called midwifery graduates or good candidates for future LDR midwives, though they are qualified with only a BSc in Nursing as far as the

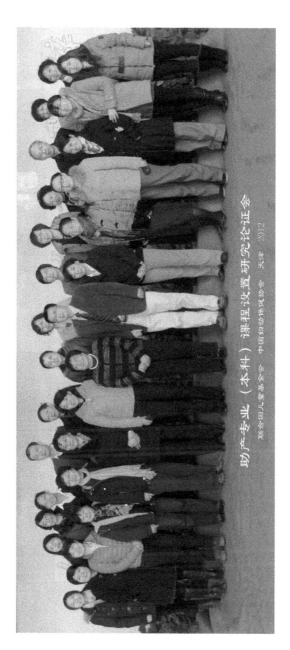

Figure 6.1 The participants of the meeting to discuss the curriculum developed for the proposed BSc degree in midwifery in *Tānjīn* Medical University

Source: Photo taken and contributed by Shouyan Yan (闫守堃).

national registration system allows. It seems to be that the national education system still has some unfinished business to complete regarding what kind of midwives and midwifery system they expect to have.

In 2016, a list of 173 colleges and universities (apart from the earlier mentioned eight key universities) advertised online midwifery courses in the BSc in nursing which they offered, from which the high school graduates were able to choose (Li 2016). It seems that the BSc in midwifery programmes are still at the planning or experimental stage or are only now organising staff training.

The absence of university-based, higher education and a standards-based curriculum for midwives makes it very difficult for them to think of and to treat pregnancy and birth as normal life events. Meanwhile, international evidence shows that higher education has raised the status and autonomy of midwives elsewhere, granting them more authority vis-à-vis medicine and nursing (De Vries et al. 2001).

Of the midwifery teaching staff, none is self-governing and responsible for developing and leading the policies and curriculum of a midwifery education programme. Furthermore, no midwifery programmes in the country take account of national and international policies and standards to meet maternity workforce needs. The contradiction between the clinical competence and theoretical teaching competence among teaching staff reveals the discrepancy between the reality and the theory. None of the midwife clinical teachers are qualified according to the ICM definition of a midwife. Worst of all is the non-existence of either a proper job description or a career ladder for midwives, which result in poor midwifery education.

Currently, midwifery is not formally recognised in China as a discipline under the present administration, with midwives being registered as either nurses or doctors and employed as such. Their job promotion pathways are subsumed either under nursing or medicine or both, leading to a dominant medical culture, increasing problem finding, unnecessary medical interventions, increasing caesarean rates and a lack of woman-centred midwifery care.

There are no midwifery schools in most provinces or in the medical universities. Although China currently does not have university-based midwifery degree programmes, it has a long history of secondary midwifery education (see Chapter 4) started in 1908. Despite the above mentioned a midwifery undergraduate programme was in the making at the University of Beijing and funded by the UNICEF. None of the teaching centres provides a framework for design, implementation and evaluation of a midwifery programme which corresponds to global expectations of competencies, accountability and education standards. The slow development of midwifery education results from the absence of a vision, a mission, a national policy, standards or employment for midwives after graduation.

In addition, few midwifery teachers have demonstrated their competence in midwifery practice, though many hold a current licence or registration to practise midwifery. The gap between their theoretical knowledge and their clinical competence is remarkable. Systematic research is much needed to overcome the absence of international standards and the inappropriately heavy emphasis on theoretical study relative to clinical practice in the education system.

The recommendations the respondents made are to establish a national midwifery education system, to establish entry criteria and a professional career ladder and to improve their pay in order to improve the basic education of midwives in China and to promote the development of education.

Absent: a regulatory framework

Despite the efforts of Chinese midwives, since 1949 there has been neither a statutory body for midwives in China to protect the public nor a professional body to educate and support midwives. In the absence of such organisations, the governmental health authorities regulate the practice of midwifery via medical legislation (see Further Reading and Notes – Midwifery policies in China). All regulations are medicine and/or nursing specific at national level. The members of the regulatory authority are not midwives reflecting the diversity of midwifery practice in the country. There is no provision for lay members or the governance structures of the regulatory authority to be set out. This puts midwifery firmly under the control of medicine.

The standard of midwifery care is seen from a medical and/or nursing perspective, obscuring standards of service in the eyes of the public. Specific legal and professional standards which midwives can use to enable them to practise in everyday situations and to pursue their continuing professional education are also non-existent. The lack of such rules, guidance and supporting services renders Chinese midwives vulnerable to accusations of malpractice and negligence.

From a Weberian point of view (Haralambos & Holborn 2008: 47–50) the medical or midwifery professions can be seen as occupational groups controlled primarily in the interests of members. This is presented, like other professions, in the form of restriction of entry into the occupation by controlling training, qualifications required for membership and the necessary period of service. The professionals' behaviour is controlled by a code of professional practice, often reinforced by law. Their skills and knowledge provide them with power which is essential for the functional well-being of the occupational group members.

Chinese midwives are a small group. They have been less able to pursue the interests of their profession than their medical colleagues (Cheung et al. 2005b; Cheung 2009) and have been gradually de-skilled as their role has been reduced (Braverman 1975). The scope of their practice is reduced to obstetricians' assistants in history taking, physical assessment, coordinating consultations, and referrals. They become nurses and doulas and have failed to achieve control over their profession and their job. They are increasingly employed in labour rooms in larger hospitals, both in rural and urban settings. They no longer play a key role in maintaining and promoting health and facilitating normal childbirth. The independence and autonomy of their profession are declining within the medically and nursing-stratified health care system.

The results of the ICM GAW tool on regulation show an absence of an officially recognised definition of a professional midwife in China. There is no legislation in China that recognises midwifery as a self-regulated profession. The cadres with midwifery skills in China are mainly obstetricians, nurses and a very small number of two/three-year trained midwives. The term *midwives* is used to refer to nurses working in labour wards and the training for these nurses to become 'midwives' is three months (Pang 2010).

The immediate regulatory authorities in China are the health care authority of each city, for example, the Department of Maternal and Child Health, Beijing Health Bureau, and the Division of Maternal and Child Health in the National Health and Family Planning Commission (discussed in Chapter 5). These governmental bodies regulate other professions at the same time, such as nurses, physicians and village health workers. There is has been no register of midwives since 2002 and no regulatory body or career ladder for midwives.

Many nurses attend women in childbirth as unqualified midwives or medical practitioners and receive no penalty. The labour and delivery room (LDR) health workers often use and are addressed by the title of doctor, and they are not guilty of an offence because of the absence of any legislation. The provision of this law should be developed urgently in order to protect the public and tackle the present dishonesty and falsification of the practitioners' titles.

Physicians are required to renew their licences every five years through a theory examination. Nurses also renew their licences every five years through a combination of a theory test and a clinical working experience certificate. As to midwives, or maternity health workers, they are subsumed under the regional management of nurses or doctors. They are re-registered as nurses or doctors every five years, audited and issued a permit of 'obstetric special technical services' every three years.

Every three years for permit renewal, LDR nurses and midwives have to attend one day in-service training before their initial registration and take part in the theory test after passing the nursing clinical competence test until they eventually become an assistant professor or assistant nursing officer. Although, on becoming an assistant professor or nursing officer they will be exempted from the examination, they still need their licence to be renewed every three years as nurses rather than midwives because the national health authority does not have a register for midwives.

The confusion in the case of Chinese midwifery is that midwifery is regulated and guided by the rules and professional organisations of both medicine and nursing.

The ICM GAW respondents were unclear if the Ministries of Health and of Education collaborated or not. Medical education programmes are accredited and managed by the Chinese Medical Association. Curriculum development and specialties require the approval of the relevant authorities of the Ministry of Education. However, midwifery education programmes did not require accreditation or approval of the government as each college designs its own educational programme.

Half of the respondents believed that the regulations in China included a scope of practice for midwives and a basic set of competencies for midwifery practice, but one of them disagreed. None of them thought these competencies, if there were any, were based on the ICM global competencies. No midwives in China can prescribe but only administer medications. However, midwives in most areas were required to be competent to perform basic emergency Obstetric and Newborn Care (BEmONC).

Considerable effort would be expected to be made by a professional body with respect to the following:

a   Regulating its own proceedings
b   Formation, maintenance and publication of the register/roll
c   Prescribing the course of training and regulating the conduct of examinations for nurses, midwives and medical practitioners
d   Organising refresher courses for practising nurses, midwives and medical practitioners
e   The issue and the form of certificate to nurses, midwives and medical practitioners and the titles which may be used and the uniforms/badges to be worn by them
f   Defining the conditions under which registered nurses, midwives and medical practitioners may be suspended from practice
g   Anything considered necessary for the purpose of making these rules effective

Lack of a national midwives association

Midwives in China have not had a national midwives association to support them and their practice since 1949, though four midwifery associations at city and provincial levels have recently found their way into existence. The lack of standards and guidance provided by their national professional organisation is one of the main reasons, in addition to the absence of a regulatory framework (as discussed in the previous section), for the decline of the profession. Chinese midwives, thus, have had to work under rules established by their medical counterparts nationally. As a result, medicine has dominated and led to the denigration and marginalisation of Chinese midwifery (Cheung et al. 2005b, 2009).

In response to this denigration and marginalisation, some discussion and experiments took place to study the relationship between midwives' roles and their responsibilities in China. Studies in *Shēnzhèn* compared the findings of 2003 with those of 1997 (Table 6.1). Although the vaginal birth rates were admirable, shocking cervical laceration rates were noted but ignored in the study, which deserves our attention.

There was not any record of perineal lacerations reported apart from no cases of third-degree perineal tears. Although the cervical laceration cases were decreased by more than half in 2003, the frequency of this occurrence still causes concern. Cervical laceration is usually caused by (mis)use of obstetric forceps and possibly vacuum extraction. These cannot be completely responsible for these injuries because the total number of such assisted births was only 100. This suggests that premature/guided pushing was routine in their midwifery practice, which might lead to cervical oedema and eventual tears. These data suggest that the midwives were alienated from their traditional midwifery skills and enslaved by their routine reliance on obstetric interventions.

This highlights the heated debate about the need to differentiate normal birth from vaginal birth in order to promote physiological birth (Downe 2008; Beech et al. 2008). The need for a professional body and a statutory body, like the UK's Royal College of Midwives (RCM) and Nursing and Midwifery Council (NMC), to regulate and promote the standard of midwifery practice to protect the public and midwives' interests, respectively, should be addressed urgently.

These problems may be associated with the revolution in maternity care having progressed so quickly. The traditional birthplace was moved from home to hospital in the 1960s in most Westernised countries (Tew 1998). China has been enthusiastic for this new development, particularly since the 1980s. That 'doctor knows best' was accepted and reflected in maternity policy (CMoH et al. 2003), with medical power sometimes seeming to be a burden to service users. Yet frequently was such confidence something of an illusion to midwifery professionals.

Midwife leaders have subsumed their ideas and practices under the opinions of obstetricians and have been steadily weaned from total, continuous non-interventionist midwifery care to acceptance of medical interventions (see Further Reading and Notes – Midwifery policies in China). They lost the interdisciplinary struggle because of the weakness of their professional and occupational organisation.

To protect mothers from treatment by incompetent midwives, a professional body and a statutory body are needed more than ever. Obstetric technology and skills are sometimes used as a source of income generation by institutions. These institutions take care to present the supremacy of medical power by projecting its

Table 6.1 Shēnzhèn: Cervical laceration rates and mode of birth

Year	Total Births	Normal Births	Suction	Forceps	Caesarean	Cervical laceration
1997	3,789	3,430	59	27	359	274	7.99%
2003	3,709	3,271	9	5	438	102	3.16%

Sources: *Xŭ* & *Wáng* (2005); *Wáng* et al. (2005).

obstetric technology and its efficacy in terms of duration of labour and precise timing of birth. With this medical supremacy, midwives were still generally held in contempt. The introduction of a national professional body would strengthen midwives' professional status and power to ensure that they support women and encourage normal physiological birth.

Midwifery as a profession in China

The examination of midwifery in China as a profession since the early 20th century is difficult, balancing what was significant then against what is significant now. Women healers and midwives alike have played a crucial role in caring for childbearing women since the 2nd century (Lee 2008: 251–3). However, midwives have rarely been mentioned as a professional group. It is difficult to find out what traditional midwives/TBAs (*chăn-pó* in history) actually did and what they were allowed or expected to do in China until the Management Rules for Traditional Birth Attendants were published in 1928 by the Chinese Ministry of the Interior (CMoI 1928; see Chapter 4).

The Midwives Rules (CMoH 1928) were developed from the European medical midwifery model, which was, albeit foreign, to provide Chinese midwives with technological aspirations for professional legitimacy. Both political and technological aspects of professional legitimacy were of primary importance in professionalisation, which had economic and social implications for midwives. In order to protect the public, the rules advocated a gradual eradication of untrained birth attendants from midwifery. They led to the development of the first register of midwives, to keep a record of those who had completed successfully its approved course of education and had the skill to practise; unfortunately this register, abolished by the government in 2001, no longer exists (CMoH 2001, 2017).

The Chinese health care system nowadays does not offer any community midwifery or nursing services. Midwives or nurse-midwives have no career ladder to achieve promotion as a midwife. This shows that investment in scaling up the midwifery workforce still has a long way to go; additionally, it must go beyond simply increasing numbers to focus on providing relevant, quality education for midwives.

The LDR nurses or midwives interviewed for this project revealed that they, after being employed, quickly mastered instrumental and operational skills, such as applying obstetric forceps and undertaking caesareans as ways of managing childbirth (as discussed in Chapter 10). Acquiring these skills made them feel good, and, to them, technology was a powerful defender of their interests in the struggle for technical change and superior status, putting them on a par with other professions. We discuss these midwives' struggle in detail in Chapter 10.

The gains of midwives in the struggle for higher status were often made at the expense of the interests of women and their newborns. Despite their efforts, midwives have remained low status and a second-class profession in the educational system (see Chapter 4). Midwifery customarily had lower entrance standards, which could well have led to the belief that midwives were imperfectly educated; as a result, in 2002, they were regarded by the state media as being no longer fit even to attend normal births (People's Daily 2001, 2002). They were poorly paid compared with their obstetric colleagues, although leading midwives might demand a slightly higher income but had little expectation of promotion. Rarely, promotion for the leaders might be achieved via the obstetric route for which they were not trained in the first place. The difficulties they faced can be imagined.

The growing importance of medical practitioners introduced bureaucratic medical structures to hospitals and clinics; these comprised examinations, organisation of health care, community approval, media pressure and so on. Under such a bureaucracy, midwives were not even allowed to offer antenatal or postnatal checks in some hospitals. The dominance of medical technology served to de-skill midwives, actively excluding them from areas of technological work.

Still, professional midwifery in modern China, as embedded in city hospital settings, was generally unwelcome. We saw villagers in central China opting for the services of traditional midwives, as mentioned in Chapter 10, and the active practice of an unlicenced traditional midwife in northern China, whose story is told in Chapter 10. The local approval of the activities of traditional midwives or birth attendants indicates that the professionalisation of midwifery cannot be realised solely in political and modern technological terms. Midwifery professionalisation in this case has social and cultural dimensions. The social dimension is the social relationships between different parties, between the service provider and the service user. The cultural dimension is the shared values in childbirth, in women, in the family and in the community in which the birth takes place. The continuous existence of traditional midwifery practice has relied heavily on these relationships and values.

Midwifery in China has remained subordinate to medicine because the professional hierarchy regards doctors as experts who possess technical knowledge and skills which midwives do not. Midwifery has never managed to become an independent profession as identified by Harris et al. (2009a). Although 'autonomy' is an essential feature of a profession according to Freidson (1970a, b, 1986), it has not survived in Chinese midwifery. The meaning of a profession is in a constant process of negotiation with others during social interactions. The implications of these various practices lead to the assumption of the lower status of Chinese midwifery within health care institutions.

Technologies and skills have been attractive to professionals because they enabled practitioners to claim to know more about women's bodies than women themselves. For example, pregnant women would believe the findings of abdominal palpation or the results of ultrasound examinations rather than their experience of the growth of the foetus.

Once technologies exist, the reliability of technological evidence may lead to insecurity and over-dependence by the professionals. This does not necessarily make women the victim of the technologies (Freidson 1970a, b, 1986; Wajcman 1993: 71). Some women like to give birth supported by high-tech interventions as, in China, they are a symbol of status or purchasing power. Women may experience a sense of greater satisfaction, control and self-empowerment than they would have if left to nature. Others, though, may feel they have become victims of technology.

In a survey about midwives' views about their own roles and abilities in a midwife-led unit in *Hángzhōu*, China, the findings suggest that midwives were confident about their practice (Cheung et al. 2009a). They still felt, though, that professionalisation of Chinese midwifery was badly needed to elucidate the place of midwives in maternity care and to replace financially motivated and interventive obstetric care in normal childbirth (James & Willis 2001; Grossman 2008).

One hundred and nine midwives (76.2% of 143) in the authors' survey in 2004 had 11 to 30 years of experience of working in LDR (Cheung et al. 2009a). The minimum duration of nursing and/or midwifery education was two years, and the maximum was more than eight years. A number of reasons were given for this. First, the system pressures them to further their education, since promotion normally goes to those with better qualifications. People with further educational qualifications are more likely to enter the posts which are functionally perceived to be more important to society, and staff are more aware of the responsibilities that such jobs entail. Another reason may be professional rivalry. Only 3 of 143 LDR nurses/midwives were working at a high managerial level, despite the fact that 38 (26.6%) of them had been trained for more than eight years and each of these 38 had over 21 years working experience in labour delivery rooms. The interviews found that the existing ranking of midwives and medical staff leads to tension between the professionals in hospitals. Although midwives are able and willing to assist with normal childbirth, they did not want to challenge medical decisions, just in case there was a legal dispute as one midwife testified:

> Why should we take more responsibilities, make no peace with our medical colleagues and put ourselves in a vulnerable position?

The industrialisation of society and use of technology indicate that medical 'experts' have increased the part they play in maternity services, and this reinforces the marginalisation of Chinese midwives. As a result Chinese maternity services can neither encourage normal birth nor acknowledge the expertise of midwives and their profession (Cheung et al. 2005b, 2006b).

For many decades there was little evidence to demonstrate any significant change in the practice of and profiles in Chinese midwifery. Nor was there much difference between the trained and untrained in their social and economic status. Midwives were increasingly viewed as part of the medical structure of care. Chinese nursing websites and advertisements in nursing journals are still associated with older symbols of nursing, such as uniforms, caps, shoes and candles, which express the desire for respectability and professional status.

Some Chinese nurse-midwives attempted to pursue collective action in order to improve their prospects, but they were minorities (Cheung et al. 2009a). The limits to their professional development were demonstrated by their lack of assertiveness to question their present practices and to challenge their social position; this was aggravated by the absence of an effective union or association of their own. As a profession, nurse-midwives should consider the practice of midwives further afield; they should also look at the availability, accessibility, acceptability and quality of the midwifery workforce and services (UNFPA et al. 2014).

Professional power and autonomy

Professionalisation entails the achievement of professional power, which carries with it autonomy (Wajcman 1993: 69); this has become a *raison d'être* for many practitioner associations. On one hand, there is a movement for governments, media, and patient groups to control and emphasise consumer protection and professional accountability, which is supposedly driven by concern for service users' interests. On the other hand, self-regulation is crucial to autonomy and enables midwives to be clear about what is expected of them and to set standards and tenets by which their practice should be measured (Lawrence & Yearley 2008: 267–8; ICM 2010, 2011a, b).

Childbearing has been treated as a medical problem in China since the 1980s when China began to open up to the outside world. The medical profession formulated maternal and child welfare policies and influenced the form and method of maternity care delivery. This was obvious in midwifery textbooks and in the routine management of hospitals. It reflected the management's belief in 'scientific' appraisal and technological interventions, as measured by efficiency and the safety of mother and newborn.

There has been growing psychological pressure to respond to the development and challenge of maternity services in the West. This was represented in the form of frequent futile visits to Western countries to observe nursing developments. There were also numerous collaborative midwifery/nursing projects between China and other countries. As most midwives were less well educated in China, they found difficulty in voicing their concerns, and even if they managed to speak up about choices and types of maternity care, their voices were suppressed or unheard.

Evidence of the increasing Western influence is found in instrumental deliveries having become the norm and caesarean rates of 100% being not unknown in China (Huang 2000). The change is driven by not only approved 'scientific' evidence but also the existence of controversies, an example of which is found in the great changes for midwives in terms of their jobs. Most of them were transformed in their maternity services into obstetricians, nurses or doulas. They were offered a choice to be nurses if working outside a LDR or to be medical doctors if working in rural areas and having received further training (Chinese Ministry of Health and Ministry of Politics 1979). The LDR nurses, who are called midwives, have been obliged to locate their practice between a medical emphasis on danger and pathology and a more traditional but easily romanticised emphasis on birth as a healthy life event. Many basic aspects of the management and care of women in labour were dictated by medical personnel or hospital policy. They were required to adhere to rules and regulations set by hospitals dominated by medical professionals. The way they managed their midwifery care was expressed in medical perceptions of childbirth and in medical attitudes towards service users. Regulation and control of professions, including medicine, are essential to safeguard public interests. The practitioners' self-esteem and the integrity of their services have been buttressed by social hierarchies and the codes of behaviour of obstetrics. This has inevitably led to the loss of midwifery identity and the disappearance of midwives (see Chapters 4 and 6).

In comparison with other professionals, midwives have been taught in schools of nursing but not universities, especially since 1949. They are employed as LDR nurses and have limited opportunities in education, in specialisation and in the status of their specialties. Therefore, they have been disadvantaged in negotiating with society. They have been driven out of offering domiciliary birth and ante-/postnatal care and into the lower professional status of doulas, nurses and people escorting women to hospital. Their profession was expected to disappear (People's Daily 2001). Their unique selling point, individualised continuity of care, is now offered by doulas instead of midwives. Midwives did not seem able to claim their professional power and status. This indicates a need for a systematic examination of the maternity services. What is required is great commitment, resources, planning and considerable tolerance in the future maternity services to narrow the difference between what women expect and what those services can offer.

Discussion: developments in midwifery

The development of Chinese midwifery is subsumed under medicine as medical personnel in China have a relatively well-functioning structure. The medical practitioners are well protected by the medically dominated health system. More unfairly, it may be argued, it serves the doctors' interests to present midwives as ignorant, dangerous and less educated. Thus power is wrongly exercised, whereby the Chinese health authorities do not or will not see the flaws of the system but, rather, blame midwives (People's Daily 2001, 2002). Chinese midwives have not been supported by appropriate professional or academic qualifications or by any midwifery professional bodies. This applies particularly in clinical practice and in education. For example, the textbooks in use still recommend routine skin preparation by shaving, enemas, episiotomy (Liu H.X 2005: 39–42) and rectal examinations every two or four hours (Kong 2005: 77–8) during labour. Teachers and textbook compilers working in the academic setting know little about the development of practice, and clinical teachers know little about the theoretical development of their profession.

However, professionalisation does not necessarily lead to a 'better' service, because it aims to protect members and to raise their status. It has also disadvantages connected with medicalisation and social control. The modern criteria of a profession (James & Willis 2001; Grossman 2008) stress extensive training, qualifications, autonomy, commitment, recognition by the state and social status. Some of these necessities are professional ideals rather than reality. Practitioners do not or could not occupy a fixed position in the social hierarchy. A person with long-term illness may have enough experience to become sceptical of certain treatments and the relationship with their practitioners. As a result, it may prove difficult for the practitioner to claim a monopoly of relevant knowledge. Another example to illustrate this point is the presence of traditional birth attendants. Despite consistent attempts to eliminate them, they act as midwives and are possibly better distributed particularly in rural areas than biomedical practitioners. This is because medical professionals prefer clustering together in and around urban areas to being scattered in rural areas.

The current role of midwives worldwide and the organisation of maternity services are changing towards providing women with increased choice and control over childbearing, and towards increased continuity of care. This means the profession is developing. However, the development of the profession has also resulted in midwifery practice becoming more hierarchical, which marginalises part-time midwives. According to some feminist writers, professionalisation in modern industrial society adopts masculine strategies, which, it can be argued, are the root of professional hierarchy (Wajcman 1993). The professional hierarchy in the development of the midwifery profession may have also adopted such strategies.

Professionalisation (Grossman 2008) of midwifery should become a process for Chinese midwives to promote normal birth. This would carry the additional benefit of consolidating their position in maternity care. As well as improving women's childbearing experience, promoting normal birth would enhance the autonomy of midwifery and midwives' control of their own occupation. Similar to other professionals elsewhere, Chinese midwives, on the whole, are working towards a higher specialisation among the health care professions.

Midwifery as a profession in China should have a distinct education system, its own statutory body and its own professional associations, philosophy and code of conduct. However, the absence of these features disables and marginalises this profession. Chinese midwives should continue to draw on their past for the purpose of reconstructing the profession and their identity. Chinese midwifery as a profession is striving to provide the services which are in the interests of the public.

Continuous redefinition of its role is a feature of a profession undergoing social change. Chinese midwifery benefits from the process of professionalisation and is becoming a profession, but at the same time it can be disadvantaged if it falls into the obstetric and technological traps. Professionalisation poses a dilemma for the midwifery profession and the public. The core of this problem is people's actions and the choices that shape their ideas about professionalisation and the technology that are so prominent in our lives.

7 Modernising childbirth in China (1928–2017 CE)

Since the 1990s, China has been growing economically and politically and becoming more modern. There is a problem, though, of determining what is 'new' and what is 'old'. The concept of 'modern' for China is generally recognised by historians as beginning from the mid-19th century, when imperial China was seriously challenged by European powers (Schurmann & Schell 1967a, b, c). It may not be coincidental that it was during this period that the concept of 'modern' also entered European intellectual life, with the emergence of up-to-date classic social theories like those of Karl Marx, Emile Durkheim and Max Weber (Barnard & Spencer 2002: 337). Modern European intellectual life and social change related directly to the Renaissance, European colonisation of other continents and the Scottish Enlightenment in the 14th, 15th and 17th centuries. If radical change is implied in what is 'modern', the concept of 'modernisation' might have been equally applied to these developments in Europe and to any other developments. Modern social theorists and historians obviously did not think so for good reason, one of which is the importance of 'time' in human conceptualisation of the world.

Indeed, 'modern' is a very convenient concept in our contemporary world – so convenient that it has become fashionable to the extent of being a 'must'. The marker of modernity is omnipresent in social, economic and political discourse in both higher and lower income countries in their efforts to change their circumstances. The changes made will provide us with an understanding of what is 'modern'.

Making sense of modernisation

Modernisation is a fashionable term in China, meaning 'the process of change initiated by industrialisation' (Macionis & Plummer 1998: 673). It was perceived as an aspiration to preserve the 'independence and sovereignty' of the country according to Fei (2007: 89–104), an influential Chinese sociologist. He acknowledged the transformations and developments connected to modernisation, and that the country on the whole had mistaken it for Westernisation. Having absorbed western technology, the Chinese were confronted with economic imbalance, social disintegration and over-medicalisation. This is particularly marked in childbearing. Obstetric 'modernisation' has caused the demise of Chinese midwifery (People's Daily 2001, 2002). That is why we discuss the issue of modernisation in this chapter.

China is a fast-developing third-world country and is searching for modernisation, a complex sociological and political issue (see Chapter 8). According to anthropologists, 'modernisation' could be regarded as a broad synonym for 'industrialisation'. This refers to a process of intellectual development motivated by 'a spirit of constant challenge to received forms or simply a process of changes' (Barnard & Spencer 2002: 376–9). Neither is static but is in the process of progression (Haralambos & Holborn 2008: 473). British sociologist Steve Bruce (2000) regards modernisation as involving 'socialisation', 'differentiation', 'rationalisation' and 'egalitarianism' (Haralambos & Holborn 2008: 446). The concept of 'modernisation' has changed people's idea about nature, which is especially true of childbirth and leads to the medical model of health (Macionis & Plummer 1998: 559). This linear 'scientific' model would allow simplification of childbearing processes and generalisations about nature and the world, leading to rejection of personal, relational, partnership-orientated, individually responsive and compassionate approaches.

Modernisation theory

The contrast between a dynamic West and a relatively static East is a part of a mode of thought that gave rise to 'modernisation theory' in the 1950s (Marsh et al. 1996: 364–5; Macionis & Plummer 1998: 306–19; Stockman 2000: 31). There is a range of modernisation theories. Most of them distinguish between 'traditional' society and 'modern' society. The former rests on customs being passed down from generation to generation, while the latter requires people to use reasoning to look into present conditions and into the alternatives for an uncertain future. In this way, people decide on social, economic and scientific developments. The emphasis on reasoning places science and technology at the core of the process of modernisation, which is attracting increasing attention in China.

Modernisation theory maintains that successful development hinges on acquiring advanced technology. An American modernisation theorist, Rostow (1960), argued the importance of developing countries overcoming obstacles to modernisation embedded in their society, for example, rejecting outdated structures, institutions and practices and stimulating mass consumption of goods and services, including social welfare (Haralambos & Holborn 2008). Traditional cultural patterns are widely perceived as the main barrier to modernisation. Such a Western, ethnocentric notion of modernisation theory was transformed as China has attempted to achieve modernisation to serve Chinese socio-economic needs since the 1980s. As a result midwifery became perceived as symbolising backwardness (as discussed in Chapters 4 and 5; People's Daily 2002).

Chinese ways of life and philosophy persist, but the conceptual framework of 'four modernisations' (of industry, agriculture, science and defence) was first put forward by the First Session of the National People's Congress (NPC) in 1954.

The framework did not become central to state policy until after 1978. China has begun to change, while respecting some traditions, ever since (Stockman 2000: 32). Such developments go beyond the development of science and technology, having brought changes in social values and ways of life.

As in many other parts of the world, one consequence of modernisation in China is the medicalisation of childbirth. In China, most urban women choose to birth in hospital, which increasingly uses technological interventions, such as induction of labour, continuous electronic fetal monitoring, epidural analgesia, amniotomy, oxytocin augmentation, episiotomy, Ventouse, forceps and caesarean. The meaning of *normal* has been expanded to embrace hospital confinement and routine unnecessary applications of technology by 'exploring social patients resources 挖掘社会病员资源' with an epidural rate of over 77% annually' in *Běijīng* (BHM-CHH 2015), regardless of the scientific evidence not supporting their routine use. It is possible that this 'exploration' is being undertaken with a view to increasing income generation. Therefore, the definition of 'normal birth' deserves attention.

Meanings of *normal birth*

Traditionally the meaning of *normal birth* in China was any birth without interventions or instrumental assistance of medicine-men or doctors. Later on, with the introduction of biomedical practice, this definition of normal birth was developed to include obstetric-assisted deliveries as well as physiological vaginal births. The latter means spontaneous births without any intervention; but the former are vaginal births with some interventions, such as induction of labour, epidural, amniotomy, augmentation and/or episiotomy. These two categories coincide with the medical designation of 'normal birth' reported in the developed world (Downe 2008; Crabtree 2008).

Recent debates around controversial areas of childbirth (Downe 2004a,b, 2008) included questions relating to 'What is normal birth?' 'What decides the acceptable knowledge of childbirth?' and 'What is the current childbirth paradigm?' Only when some Chinese midwives defined their areas of practice in the development of the first 'Midwife-led' Homely Birth Unit in China, did they become aware of these debates and the need for introducing a third category of 'obstetric delivery' into Chinese midwives' vocabulary (see Chapter 5). This term was proposed by the UK-based Association for Improvements in the Maternity Services (AIMS) (Beech 2008: 70). 'Obstetric delivery' comprises a vaginal delivery preceded by a variety of interventions, such as artificial rupture of the amniotic membranes, induction or acceleration of labour, epidural anaesthesia and/or episiotomy. As a result, the meaning of 'normal birth' needs to be modified.

The World Health Organization defines normal birth as

> spontaneous in onset, low risk at the start of labour and remaining so throughout labour and delivery. The infant is born in the vertex position between 37 and 42 completed weeks of pregnancy. After birth mother and infant are in good condition.

(WHO 1999a)

This definition does not exclude a range of interventions and instruments being used. Therefore, the dichotomy of normal and operative deliveries still remains here as the predominant categories for the definition of childbirth (Beech 2008) and the definition of normal birth is yet to be explored and redefined.

Medical intervention has been justified on the grounds that it saves lives, and yet, there has been no corresponding fall in maternal or perinatal deaths (Beech & Phipps 2008). Many Chinese health workers are not fully aware that the proliferation of 'normality' should not lead to the rejection or devaluation of science and technology but to promotion of a humanistic, non-interventionist and holistic midwifery paradigm (Davis-Floyd et al. 2009).

Medicalisation of childbirth

Childbirth has always been an important event in human life. The focus of feminist medical historians has been on the role of women healers and midwives (Ehrenreich 1976; Donnison 1988). A male-dominated western medical profession emerged during the 18th century, giving men increasing control over the birth process and obstetric technology in determining the outcome. The professionalisation discussed in Chapter 6 has brought more intervention in childbirth and attracted criticism from leading practitioners and scholars (Donnison 1988; Wajcman 1993).

The concept of modernisation has been advanced by critics of modern medicine and medical sociologists (Illich 1975; Oakley 1980, 1987; Haralambos & Holborn 2008: 291). 'Iatrogenesis' was identified by Illich (1975) as resulting from medical intervention. In childbirth, the technocratic model of birth influences attitudes and behaviours among medical practitioners (Davis-Floyd et al. 2009). This philosophical simplicity of medicalisation has profound effects on the way that 'scientific' knowledge is perceived and framed (Downe 2008: 9). Science and technology can be broken down into small building blocks, and childbirth becomes, as a result, regulated by protocols and guidelines. By this logic, the socially constructed knowledge of childbirth has been transformed into norms in terms of length of labour and statistical averages in midwifery and obstetric textbooks. This is obvious in Chinese obstetrics and midwifery (Kong 2005; Liu H.X 2005). Women's bodies have, thus, become simple birthing machines that can be controlled by average times and rules.

The medicalisation of childbirth not only affects female midwives but also increases the powerlessness of women giving birth. Along similar lines, childbirth has been moved from the domestic to institutional sphere with science and technology (Oakley & Houd 1990). Therefore, the original birthing culture has been changed, which is especially true in most Chinese hospitals nowadays. Women are having their pubic hair shaved, having their bowels emptied by enemas, lying flat on their backs and undergoing routine episiotomy. They are delivered in hospital deprived of social and family support.

The hospital has become a symbol of advanced technology, a site of power and a place of medical control involving obstetric technology and pharmacological analgesia. The maternity regulations of the state (CMoH et al. 2003) have removed women from their homes and damaged family functioning in the course of modernisation of birth. They have also transformed midwives' roles to become obstetric nurses and doulas in urban areas and to become obstetricians elsewhere and from attending birth to escorting women to hospitals. Hospitals' concerns have focused on the satisfaction of the institution and health workers, rather than of women.

The health care system has demonstrated the emergence of social control, medicalisation and bureaucracies. Medical bureaucracies have come to dominate the hierarchies of health care systems. The early 20th century saw the consolidation of hospitals, the exclusion of traditional midwives and the intrusion of medical values into numerous areas of human reproduction and people's lives. Hospitalisation of childbirth has dramatically increased birth interventions with nearly 100% caesarean rates being no longer unknown in China (Huang 2000). This development leads to calls for the return of childbirth to nature in China and the development of midwife-led care in the 21st century, based on understandings of the global birthing culture (Cheung et al. 2009a, b; Mander et al. 2009; Cheung & Fleming 2011).

This does not necessarily mean that birthing women are hostile to increased technical interventions; some technology has undeniably been of physical benefit and, in some cases, life-saving. Many women may expect more obstetric technology (Wajcman 1993: 71) as they may feel that technology offers them confidence, more choices, and 'a sense of greater control and self-empowerment' than leaving childbirth to nature (Petchesky 1987; Stanworth 1987; Wajcman 1993; Downe 2007). This viewpoint has been under-emphasised in feminist literature. From this perspective, the feminist critique goes no further than demanding access to knowledge and education so that women can make their decisions according to their own understanding (Wajcman 1993: 61).

Increased and routine technological interventions have thus gradually led to over-dependence on obstetric technology, and the supremacy of modern obstetrics, which emphasises the sick role, over midwifery (Parsons 1951; Macionis & Plummer 1998: 568–9). Routine obstetric intervention explains women's apparent tolerance of a system that, some have argued, has transformed birth into a passive and alienating experience (Donnison 1988; Wajcman 1993). Some critiques, particularly feminists', challenge modern, hospital-based obstetric practices for distancing women from their own bodies and for removing any control over the birth from women. They view the process of obstetric intervention as the loss of women's power and control to create a dehumanised birth process.

Sara Nettleton (2001) contends that a new sociological imagination of 'bodies' has been carved out by some sociologists from women's attempts to wrest control over their bodies and childbirth from male-dominated professionals. In this mind–body connection debate, the boundaries and borders of bodies, minds and spirits with nature and technology have dissolved. The biological entity of 'body' is transformed in the process of social action, technological renovation and people's understanding. It becomes a social and biological issue, and the well-being of women is shaped by culture and the definition and behaviour of society (Macionis & Plummer 1998: 574; Haralambos & Holborn 2008: 98; Davis-Floyd et al. 2009).

The concept of this 'modernisation' dominates the Chinese social 'scientific' understandings of human reproduction, which often conveys a misleading and partial picture and privileges developments in obstetric techniques rather than midwifery (Cheung 2009). Medical intervention in childbirth is perceived as a symbol of 'modernisation' (Mander 2007) in Chinese maternity care, and physiological vaginal births have gone out of fashion. This leads to the failure of health practitioners to understand the power of normal physiology in birth and the power of the mother's emotions to affect the progress of labour. Such failure continues to underlie the propensity of Chinese minds to rely on obstetric technology for physiological childbirth (CMoH et al. 2003).

Midwifery development in modern China

China progressed in recovering from the disastrous effects of the Great Cultural Revolution of 1966–1976, embarking on the 'four modernisations' (as discussed earlier) after 1976. To achieve all these goals, China had to develop greatly in science and technology. In order to make the country into one of the best in the world, thousands of students were sent abroad to study science and technology, including medicine. They returned with 'new concepts' of science and technology.

Soon after these ideas were introduced, midwifery was captured and nearly controlled by obstetricians and obstetric technology. In practice many obstetricians, especially the less-experienced, were incompetent in normal birth because they had no experience of normality. They frequently employed instruments unnecessarily to accelerate the birth and save their time (Huang 2000). Thus, technology was crucial for obstetricians in determining the outcome of labour. They became reluctant to make clinical judgements on the basis of their own abilities and experience, relying on non-evidence-based protocols and hospital regulations.

This process of birthing management has converted childbirth into a medical problem (Macionis & Plummer 1998: 571). Women have given birth without medical help for centuries, but, although this remains true in many rural areas, it no longer holds in urban China, where various degrees of medical intervention are routine. Childbirth is no longer a family event predicted on the basis of knowledge about human biological functioning. The bodies of women have become enslaved to obstetric technology and childbirth is firmly controlled by the social institution of medicine.

In recent years, China has been undergoing social transition towards a more market-led economy. Obstetric technology has unfortunately become manageable and cost-effective in the 21st century as more goods are manufactured (Cheung et al. 2005a, b, 2006a, b). The notion of normal childbirth was extended to embrace obstetric or instrumental delivery for the convenience of resource management. Medical practitioners have recognised the potential of the greater use of obstetric technology, which has been further extended by the development of new forms of analgesia, anaesthesia, antisepsis, asepsis and operative techniques.

Modernisation should not be blamed for causing all social problems. Such a patriarchal society does not think highly of women's intelligence, so the gender of Chinese women and midwives places them in a vulnerable position. In health care, they could not escape the same awful fate. Care is also governed by supply and demand, such as when privatised hospitals try to balance their books; they explore the maternity services and the medicalisation of birth to increase profit and power.

The turn of the millennium in China witnessed a radical change in the perception of other countries' obstetric technology. Total hospitalisation of childbirth was promoted following the example of developed countries in the 1970s (CMoH et al. 2003). In *Běijīng* 100% caesarean rates were reported (as discussed in Chapters 4 and 8) and obstetricians' claims to be experts in the modernisation of childbirth have brought to public attention the problem of medicalisation (Huang 2000). In response, a growing social awareness has called for something to be done about the problem (Cheung et al. 2006a; Souza et al. 2010; Feng et al. 2012).

Science and obstetric technology have dominated people's thoughts and imagination, despite the female body being perfectly well designed to give birth. Reproduction is crucial for the continuation and survival of the human race and is culturally defined. Childbirth has more and more become controlled by modern obstetric technology in industrial societies. Under such circumstances, many medical sociologists have argued that people should take control of their own bodies (Illich 1975; Oakley 1980) and that birthing should be personalised (Davis-Floyd et al. 2009).

Modernisation attempts in Chinese midwifery

A series of studies by the authors since 2004 have shown that technological interventions in normal childbirth became routine, changing women's birthing experience (Cheung & Pan 2012). Hospitalisation of childbirth in China was seen to indicate an advanced standard of care (CMoH et al. 2003). Because midwifery was enshrined in tradition, Chinese midwifery has been brushed aside in this framework of modernisation of childbirth (as discussed in Chapter 8; People's Daily 2001, 2002).

Whether we see the decline of Chinese midwifery as progress or as a retrograde development depends on our underlying values. In China, medical interventions present themselves as cardinal forms of 'modernisation' of childbirth in a controversial trend to replace normal vaginal birth, because they are perceived as safer and more efficient in terms of resource management. However, they separate the mind from the body and redefine the body as a machine that can be repaired medically, with birthing women as their objects and patients.

According to the vision and mission of midwives set by the International Confederation of Midwives, the process of modernisation of childbirth should ensure 'every woman has access to a midwife's care', and midwives should be 'the most appropriate caregivers for childbearing women and in keeping birth normal, in order to enhance the reproductive health of women, and the health of their new-borns and their families' (ICM 2017).

In a global context, the definition of modernisation has, thus, become increasingly problematic and open to empirical critique.

Hospital-based midwifery care was actually introduced into China in the late 19th century by missionaries (see Chapter 3). This has yet to be changed to normality-focused care, so as to reduce caesarean and instrumental deliveries. To do this, current Chinese midwives have to fight a steep uphill battle to establish their profession as a legitimate component in the practice of maternity care. In this regard, normality-based midwifery has been seen as a paradigm of the struggle towards modernisation of childbirth. It has involved questions about the role of midwives, their education and the application of their knowledge to the public maternity services.

In mainland China from 1928 onwards an increasing number of midwives graduated from the midwifery schools, which gave them opportunities to work in hospitals and/or formal health establishments. Because of a serious shortage of female obstetricians, many of the midwives took obstetricians' places to use obstetric technology and instruments, for example, augmentation of labour, amniotomy to shorten labour and episiotomy and forceps; they eventually became obstetricians themselves. One way to analyse this transformation is as a continuum related to modernisation. At either end of this continuum are traditional cultures of power struggle between these two professions and between these two different kinds of philosophies. This transformation of cultures is based on the 2004 government document – 'The methods for the management of midwifery and obstetric technology in *Běijīng*' (*Běijīng* Health Authority 2004) – and is also reflected in a survey distributed by the Chinese Ministry of Health in 2008 (CMoH 2008a).

The midwifery model

Midwifery models of care have been reported in Canada (MacDonald & Bourgeault 2009), Netherlands (De Vries et al. 2009), New Zealand (Hendry 2009) and Samoa (Utumuu 2009). However, it is argued that the 'midwifery model' works in childbirth in the same way that the medical model does. Midwives practise in a tension between the medical emphasis on danger and pathology and a traditional emphasis on birth as a normal life event. The healthy emphasis may be overtaken by the medical emphasis, as has happened to Chinese midwives, as their profession is marginalised, being phased out and replaced by obstetric nurses, doulas and obstetricians, as a result of medicalisation of childbirth (as discussed earlier in this chapter).

Midwifery models of care adopt a holistic approach and value the inseparability of the mothers' body, mind and spirit, and the importance of their emotions and intuition (Davis-Floyd et al. 2009). This humanistic approach is also called a social model, and post-modern model of care with slightly different emphases.

Woman-friendly and family-centred, it embodies values, ethics, philosophy, cultural appropriateness and sensitivity. The midwifery model of care facilitates autonomy and continuity of care and carer.

The focus of midwifery models is on health promotion with the active involvement and shared responsibility of birthing women and families in decision-making affecting their health and well-being (CMoH et al. 2003). The model of care is based on mutual trust and respect between midwives and women and promotes informed choice. It shows respect for human dignity and empowers women and their families to make choices through education and anticipatory guidance and role modelling. One of the hallmarks of the midwifery model of care is to provide individualised care to women, with timely referral to other health professionals when and if the client's condition warrants such transfer.

The model of continuity of midwives and midwifery care seems to be able to maximise individualised satisfaction both for birthing women and their carers. This is known as 'caseload' midwifery (Murphy-Black 1992: 113; Walsh, 2007a, b; Tracy 2007; NICE 2007), a combination of continuity of care and carers. The ideology of caseload midwifery is regarded as part of professionalisation within midwifery to regain professional autonomy, status and job satisfaction that have been eradicated by working in a hierarchical setting dominated by obstetrics (Sandall et al. 2013). Some retrospective studies in midwifery indicate that caseload midwifery care, such as the Albany practice, has benefits for women in terms of providing advice and emotional support (Edwards 2010; Homer et al. 2017).

Autonomy and continuity of carer were the best predictors of midwives' job satisfaction in a study of midwives in Aberdeen (Hundley 1995). The team continuity of care claimed by midwives may not necessarily give greater choice and control for women who have to rely on midwives' expertise. The assumption that a female dominated midwifery service is able to provide more 'women-centred' care (House of Commons Health Committee 1992; Phillips 2009) is still in need of systematic examination and evidence.

After three years of preparatory efforts, the first midwifery-led unit was developed in *Hángzhōu* to provide woman-centred care and to promote normal birth and midwifery (see Chapter 5; Mander et al. 2009; Cheung et al. 2011a, b; Pan & Cheung 2011). This development recognised that the efforts of midwives to achieve professional power and status may produce an unequal relationship between obstetricians and the mothers (Sandall et al. 2013). To achieve 'women-centred care' requires midwives to give up some of their autonomy and job satisfaction in order to create an equal relationship with women. This requires considerable commitment, resources, planning and tolerance from the professionals. Continuity constitutes a major task to improve maternity services by narrowing the difference between what women expect and what providers can offer.

Inter-professional rivalries

Childbirth presents a picture of a struggle to claim a control over childbirth between obstetricians and midwives, each representing different societal interests in birth. Tension between professions is a persistent fact, which is aggravated by the development of obstetric technology. Advances in technology and modernisation of childbirth may offer advantages but certainly give no guarantee of improving relationships between midwives and obstetricians.

Since the start of the 20th century, midwives' practice and education have been regulated, initially by medical professionals and subsequently by other bodies, such as nurses (Mander 2008). Increased midwifery specialisation has resulted from greater centralisation of services (Murphy-Black 1992: 114). Midwifery care has been divided chronologically according to different stages of childbearing. They have shaken off the lower status of birth attendants, handy-women and untrained helpers, and are said to enjoy more respect, greater independence and freedom in offering home births, where permitted.

The division between the areas of competence and responsibility is often not clear-cut. A large grey area has given rise to conflict between the expectations and practice of care and demands flexibility from all parties. Thus, midwives are expected to possess the attributes of flexibility, cheerfulness, sympathy and empathy in addition to high ethical standards (Towler & Bramall 1986: 247). The limitations of midwives' autonomy have become more apparent in large hospitals with many aspects of management being decided by medical personnel or hospital policy, for example, type of analgesia. Increasing medicalisation of childbirth has led to specialisation or fragmentation of midwifery care (DoH 1993: 38).

The medical profession has struggled to remain supreme in the administration of public health and health education. Their pressure groups have sought legislation to control midwives for the sake of medical interests, such as rights to prescribe and rights to discharge; while middle-class midwives have been seeking independent professional status. Medicine has thus become a symbolic system, expressing some basic values, beliefs and moral concerns of society, for example, the utilisation of technology or surgery to represent modernisation in maternity services.

Medical professionals were legitimated as healers and, likewise, their enthusiasm for technology. Obstetrics has always been more than a system of scientific ideas and practices; its emphases were not only on objectivity, numerical measurements and scientific rationality but were also supported by physiochemical data and reductionism. Gradually obstetricians obtained higher social status and high earning power. However, there is no such thing as uniform scientific obstetrics (Helman 2000: 82), as in each country it is practised differently because childbearing has always been essentially culture-bound.

It is now widely acknowledged (Illich 1975; Jordan 1993; Mander 2007) that many technological interventions in childbirth are unnecessary: high-risk births are probably the exception. Rather, technology reflects the powerful decision-making role of obstetricians. High intervention rates, especially in urban areas, and the misuse of instruments are still common enough to attract criticism from the public and professionals. However, in recent decades, there has been some feminist agitation in favour of caesarean and the use of anaesthesia during labour (Wajcman 1993: 71). Some regard caesarean and anaesthesia as the most advanced techniques available for women to experience quick and painless childbirth; thus, some have called for women's right to have these interventions available on demand (Sheldon & Thomson 1998).

Caesarean and anaesthesia were initially developed for saving lives but have served to increase human control over childbirth. Paradoxically, they helped change the definition of childbirth and move childbirth from a domestic event to a medical procedure only available in hospital. This wrongly perceived 'modernisation' of childbirth, such as happened in China, is described by some Western feminist authors as a kind of 'sociology' of childbirth (Oakley 1980; Wajcman 1991). These studies show ways to investigate what happens, why and with what consequences to women having babies in this medical culture.

The place of birth has also become the focus of a power struggle. The hospitalisation of birth has been an effective means to reduce the power and status of midwives as independent practitioners because they must work under the direct supervision of an obstetrician. This strengthens medical ascendancy over midwives as professional rivals (Tew 1990: 7). The introduction of midwife-led facilities is used by midwives to reclaim their status, autonomy and power. Evidence to support and quantify midwives' claims is plentiful (Campbell & Macfarlane 1996; Campbell 1997: 10).

The relationship between doctors and midwives is recognised to be highly charged and traditionally antagonistic by some qualitative studies (Ehrenreich 1976; Towler & Bramall 1986; Donnison 1988). Negotiation and bargaining about the roles have been continuing throughout history and up to the present time. Many disputes take place over the classification of the territory between 'normal' and 'abnormal' childbearing. The definition of midwives' 'normal birth' is political and implies a specific professional orientation. It assumes all pregnancies and births to be normal until proved otherwise. This approach assumes the responsibility of midwives, and it is for them to decide when to involve medical personnel. The medical model assumes that all pregnancies and births are potentially pathological until proved not (Wagner M 1994: 30). This approach assumes medical responsibility for childbearing. The 'natural' interpretation of *normal* was thought by Kitzinger (1990: 153) to be used to justify women's and midwives' resistance to medical interventions.

Professional rivalry has not been limited to the contest between midwifery and medical professions (Tew 1990: 7). Some writers argue that the increasing use of sophisticated technology is a defensive behaviour because of their exposure to crossfire from clients and colleagues. Thus, defensiveness prepares for the threat of litigation should an unfavourable outcome occur.

Holistic approaches in midwifery can bridge and balance the disparities between midwives and birthing women because of the midwives' sensibility and their historic interest in women's well-being (Page 1988: 251–2). Ideas about what women and professionals have wanted of maternity services have changed over time. What has remained constant and essential is the difference between women's perception and demands and medical preferences and priorities (Lewis 1990: 16).

Constructing normal childbirth

Our world is experienced and understood differently, depending on environment, society and culture, and our perceptions are a product of mental processes, which are culturally shaped (Barnard 2000; Barnard & Spencer 2002). Thus, defining the meaning of *normal childbirth* is challenging to midwives and sociologists because of the complexity and uncertainty of the culture in which it happens (Crabtree 2008; Downe 2008). Normal childbirth is defined differently by interested organisations such as the UK Royal College of Midwives and the National Childbirth Trust. But in China, it means all vaginal births, except instrumental deliveries.

'Active management' and 'cost-effectiveness' in hospitals lead to the development of an industrial model to increase efficiency; they also aim to decrease the uncertainty surrounding childbirth. This model means a simplification of labour management and heavy reliance upon 'high-tech' approaches in our daily construction of health risk, but this is, in fact, promoting a pathological orientation. As a result, health workers formulate certain procedures, skills or knowledge to address constrained uncertainty when caring for any single childbearing woman. Therefore, the unpredictability and complexity of childbirth are reduced to a simple linear routine of labour management, the so-called modernisation of childbirth management.

Discussion

In this chapter we have examined the meanings of normal childbirth in the context of the modernisation of childbirth in China. However, the modernisation of childbirth is elusive, since childbirth has been part of a traditional way of life for thousands of years. Still, modernisation needs to be critically scrutinised, as it is extremely challenging to write about it. The contemporary preoccupation with obstetrics and interventions has not yet led to the modernisation of childbirth in China.

The modernisation of childbirth, in a real sense, should make it more humane and holistic rather than technological in caring for healthy childbearing women. Modernisation should offer sustainable ways to empower women to improve the physiological, psychological and social outcomes of childbearing, which would be financially feasible for all families and health systems. This understanding was eventually brought to the attention of the National Health and Family Planning Commission of the People's Republic of China (NHFPC) after the ICM Gap Analysis Workshop in 2014. The NHFPC then commissioned a midwifery undergraduate education project in eight key universities and nine hospitals to set up standardised training bases for midwives (see Chapter 5). In order to speed up the training of midwives in the central and western provinces of China, the NHFPC has also been planning a programme for 5,000 nurses to prepare them to become midwives there (Pang 2016). This is clearly an important measure to promote the development of midwifery in China.

8   The marginalisation of Chinese midwives

In the 1980s Donnison observed that childbirth was generally perceived as being safer in hospital than at home (1988: 190–209), and safest in consultant units, even though statistical analysis of the data does not support this conclusion (Tew 1998). Since then, centralisation of maternity care in consultant units has become common with obstetrical technology and more specialised staff engaging in 'active management' of labour. A decade later China caught up with these developments without questioning their validity or credibility. Dr Huang (2000), a consultant obstetrician in *Běijīng*, found in her research that specialisation and overutilisation of high-tech approaches to childbirth led to the disappearance of birth units in small hospitals and to 100% caesarean rates. High-tech obstetric units have contributed to the demise of Chinese midwifery, turning midwives into obstetricians' assistants and keepers of medical equipment (see Chapter 5; Cheung et al. 2005b). If we look into history, we can see that long before the 20th century, most Chinese women were attended in labour by their elderly female neighbours, relatives or birth attendants, also called traditional midwives (*chǎn-pó*; see Chapters 3 and 4. Only the families of the emperor's family, his officers in the palace or in his government offices turned to literate and/or skilled birth attendants or traditional midwives (*wěn-pó*) or medical women (*nǚyī*), who charged for their services or received payment in kind (Furth 1987: 17; Leung 2000: 122–5; Lee 2003). Thus, women's birthing experiences differed due to differences in carers.

It cannot be denied that Chinese midwives had long provided supportive maternity care for healthy women. The meaning of midwifery care, however, was misunderstood with the increasing hospitalisation of childbirth (CMoH et al. 2003). Midwives together with traditional midwives attended more than 90% of childbearing women, but now they have been evicted from their jobs in China, particularly in urban areas. At present, more than half of their clients undergo surgery performed by obstetricians. Caesareans have become fashionable, a symbol of technological modernisation and an alternative way of birthing (Mander 2007). Chinese midwives have been transformed into obstetric nurses, doctors and doulas. Their marginalisation is something that midwives have experienced periodically in history. The more severe their marginalisation is, the more likely they are to be keenly aware of their surroundings and to question what is taken for granted.

The examination of these marginalities raises challenging questions about how margins and boundaries come about.

Historically, the terms used to describe midwives are quite confusing and potentially misleading. Their ascribed social status was the lowest of the low in Chinese social classification of *sāngū liùpó* (see Chapter 3; Guide – Chinese glossary). From its social function there is nothing to justify their low ranking and poor social position in this hierarchical society. These traditional midwives enjoyed a certain autonomy.

The part that traditional midwives played in the history of childbearing has been obscured in popular thought with the development of modern obstetric technology. Criticisms of traditional midwives from biomedically-educated doctors and midwives included their illiteracy, unscientific approach *xiàdì zùocáo* (giving birth on grass) and absence of asepsis.

The differences between traditional and biophysiological midwives are the former adopt holism, while the latter adopt linear biomedical approaches. The major disparity between them lies in their attitudes towards obstetric technology and the provision of supportive midwifery care. The biophysiological approach focuses on a diagnostic hypothetic-deductive thinking and the utilisation of modern technologies, while the traditional approach focuses on accumulated culturally orientated understanding of health and disorders.

With the aid of modern technology, biomedical Chinese midwives had nearly replaced traditional midwives in urban areas in the 20th century because science was believed to be a supreme value and a symbol of modernity (see Chapter 7). Unfortunately, by the 21st century midwives are on the verge of extinction (as discussed later in this chapter) because of the wide acceptance of medicalised childbirth.

Questions about reasons, values and their implications are the focus of this discussion. It is hoped that this book will serve as a starting point for further work in this field with more specific attention to the present development of Chinese midwifery.

Midwife–nurse relations

Although women's bodies are designed to give birth unaided, women in many societies have felt the need for a helper or companion to support them during the birth. This was usually a female relative, friend or neighbour in China as childbirth is perceived as women's business. It is similar to what happened in the West when they learned their skills from personal childbearing experience and from working alongside other birth attendants (Donnison 1988; Tew 1998: 41).

At the beginning of the 20th century in China, midwifery began to advance in the direction of the present medical model. Since then, especially in the recent decade, midwives have been wrongly blamed for high maternal and neonatal mortality, which more likely involved medical doctors and other medical professionals (People's Daily 2002). Midwives' job of caring for healthy childbearing women was reallocated to obstetric nurses and obstetricians (DHPCMH 2007).

Chinese midwives were re-classified as nurses and their associations and were merged into the Chinese Nursing Association (CAN) despite their having established the *Běipíng* Midwives Association in 1933, the Midwives Association of China in 1941 and the *Chóngqìng* Midwives Association in 1946. Midwives felt disadvantaged and handicapped by their inability to voice their unique concerns through the CAN and to advance their members' interests.

Instead of taking advantage of their association with nurses, midwives tried consistently to extricate themselves from it. Chinese midwives' leaders attended the International Confederation of Midwives (ICM) on three successive occasions. They were just observers seeking to join, hoping to learn something and get some support from ICM as they did not have their own association. Finally, in 2008, the first Midwives Association, an affiliate of the *Zhèjiāng* Nurses' Association, was established in response to the threat to midwives' roles (ZMA 2008). Founded voluntarily by midwives in *Zhèjiāng* Province, the association is a non-profit organisation that helps to promote midwifery development. Its aims are to define rules and standards locally for midwives, to promote and protect women's health, to improve newborns' health and to provide high-quality service and effective personal care. It functions like a trade union, but it is also intended to have an educational purpose and to serve the public interest. It is the first member of the ICM from mainland China, but any benefits of this membership are not yet clear.

Although they have their own association, *Zhèjiāng* midwives found difficulty extricating themselves from affiliate status to the Nurses' Association. This was because of its links through finance, personnel and political ideology, and there were concerns about the survival of this midwives association. While seeking to detach themselves from the Nurses' Association, the midwives simultaneously sought to take advantage of governmental subsidies to the Nurses' Association to ensure the sustainability of their own association.

The first much-sought-after legislation finally became the Nurses Act in January 2008, taking effect in May 2008, having been first drafted in 1985 for both nurses and midwives (CSC 2008). It would take more time for the framework to function and to develop.

The relationship between midwives and nurses is a reluctant one, on the part of midwives, as a result of the Chinese Ministry of Health policies. The policy-makers were unable to recognise the different roles of midwives, doctors and nurses in their own spheres. This approach is reflected in the governmental policies regarding maternal and child care (Further reading and notes – Midwifery policies in China, Table 3.2). To simplify organisation, they placed midwifery and nursing under the control of medicine and then replaced medical control of midwifery with control by nurses.

The denigration of midwifery

First of all, medical internal stratification and patriarchy diminished the status and development of midwifery in China. The stereotype of 'ignorant midwives' was commonplace, just like the image of low IQ and untrained nurses (People's Daily

2002). By the end of the 20th century, Chinese midwives had no choice but to attend births in labour rooms or become nurses.

Second, during dramatic social and ideological change initiated by technological modernisation and economic growth, research into Chinese midwifery has been unable to obtain funding. The lack of systematic study into the development of midwifery has resulted in midwives' inability to persuade policy-makers of the importance of providing midwifery care for women.

Third, health authorities sought, erroneously, to limit the costs of the maternity services by every conceivable means, including restructuring. This resulted in the manipulation of the meaning and practice of the doula (see Chapter 5) and an excessively heavy reliance on obstetricians and instrumental deliveries (see Chapter 7).

Fourth, proper midwifery care has not been regarded by the health authorities as a science and an art, but as backward, unprofitable and disposable. As a result, midwives were summarily replaced by obstetric nurses, doulas and obstetricians. Thus, many childbearing women have been prevented from accessing the appropriate attention. This unjustified replacement is either an indefensible position or an indefensible claim to economies.

The emergence of a cadre of highly educated and vocal midwives as a professionalising pressure group led to efforts over the last decade to develop undergraduate midwifery education and a midwife-led normal birth unit (see Chapter 5). On one hand, this struggle was between medical pressure groups seeking legislation to control midwives in their own interests, while, on the other hand, midwives were seeking independent professional status. This power struggle has involved negotiation, medical politics and the manipulation of reality (Dirks et al. 1994).

Policy development and midwifery

Being backward-looking, Chinese policy-makers had little idea of the advances made in midwifery (see Further Reading and Notes – Midwifery policies in China). Supported by government policy in 1993, the superiority of medically dominated health workers' thinking; they came to believe that Chinese midwifery was not good enough and abolished midwifery education in urban areas. As a result, the maternity services could neither keep up with the modernisation of ideas and practices nor with population growth.

Governmental policy regarding Chinese midwifery has undergone five different historical stages. They are the untroubled, idle, inactive, demise and 'midwife' a symbol of its profession.

Untroubled (700 BCE–1957)

Traditional Chinese midwifery developed unnoticed until part of it was transformed into biomedical midwifery to protect mothers from treatment by supposedly incompetent midwives. Chinese Midwives Rules were developed and introduced by the Nationalist government in 1928 (CMoHNG 1928; see

Chapter 4). The standards set were similar to those in the West, being acceptable to obstetricians. De-registration was the ultimate penalty, which was supposed to deter unqualified practitioners from offering a service deviating from officially accepted standards, when regarded as not in the mother's best interests.

A new midwifery education system was finally established by the state-run midwifery school in 1929, comprising elementary, undergraduate, and postgraduate levels (see Chapter 4). This system changed after the communists came to power in 1949. It was transformed in 1952 (Mei 1983; Gu 2004) to elementary and secondary levels only, which meant the education, could vary from several weeks to two or three years (see Chapter 4). There was no longer any undergraduate midwifery programme (Xinhua telecommunication 1951). Midwifery education was changed to normally last for two years, after six years of compulsory education, because the Chinese government considered the intermediate level was sufficient to meet the need of family-building enterprises.

There were two types of midwifery teacher training after 1952: either one year or three to six months' clinical training after at least two years' work experience. Such a midwifery educational model resulted in a social perception of midwives as second-class health workers and their service as being less trustworthy than obstetricians' (Cheung et al. 2011c). Thus, there is no evidence to show that phasing out midwifery higher education has benefited China.

Prior to the Great Leap Forward (1957), though there was no specific regulation for bio-medical midwives, their practice was covered by regulations for medical health workers (CMoH 1952; see Further Reading and Notes – Midwifery policies in China, Table 3.2). Meanwhile, traditional midwives carried out their business as usual, despite having been repressed more severely throughout China.

Idle period: biomedical midwifery (1958–1965)

In 1958 the Great Leap Forward (GLF) was launched, aiming to increase food and industrial production simultaneously. Communist leaders established agricultural collectives and then communes comprising 4,000 to 5,000 families each. Each commune was directed by political leaders answerable to the government. But the communes were impersonal and too large to be efficient. In addition, bad weather and floods damaged crops and the typical GLF's proneness to boasting and exaggeration of the achievements resulted in the 1959 famine.

In public health, a health centre was built in each commune, leading to primary health organisations mushrooming. Between 1952 and 1959 the number of maternal-child-care centres increased from 2,379 to 4,179 but with insufficient properly trained health workers (NBoSoC 1996a). The Great Leap Forward ended in failure.

Faced with these setbacks, Chinese leaders slowed the pace of industrial growth, decreased the number of the maternal-child care centres and dismissed peasant health workers in 1962. Because of such turmoil, no obvious changes occurred in Chinese midwifery and midwives' roles or in midwifery policies during this period (Further Reading and Notes – Midwifery policies in China).

Inactivity (1966–1977)

In 1966, the Great Proletarian Cultural Revolution was started. Universities and schools were closed, with midwifery schools being no exception. University students and teachers were sent to the countryside to work on farms alongside peasants. Young people, having been told they were the future for a better China, attacked teachers, party officials and others. The Cultural Revolution was eventually out of control, but Chinese midwifery was of no concern because the country was in political turmoil. In the 1970s, more than half of the national health care was provided by over 1,600,000 barefoot doctors (untrained or semi-trained) and the rest was cared for by less than 1,020,000 medically-trained and traditional Chinese medicine doctors and over 64,875 midwives (Table 8.1) and traditional midwives in the country (NBoSoC 1996b, 2002; Chapter 11).

Marginalisation (1978–2015)

An 'open-up' policy was implemented in China after the Cultural Revolution. Modernisation became the focus of the Ministry of Health (National Department 1979). Relationships among hospitals were changed from collaboration to full-scale, profit-focused and competitive. A private health care model was gradually established to encourage competition within the public sector (National Department 2005). Because midwives did not need to use modern obstetric machinery to provide care, they were denied the opportunity to attain a secure licence and mandate to practise and disappeared for more than a decade in the national health statistics (NBoSoC 1996b; 2017). The maternal-childcare institutions were reduced to 2,724 in 1998 (NBoSoC 2002). Such legal status and privileges were awarded to obstetricians and nurses. As a result, midwives were marginalised, and women and their families were unable to access midwifery services.

The regulation of Chinese midwifery has not developed well since 1949 when the present government came to power. Health policies have prevented the profession from developing, leading to the wide use of caesarean as an alternative mode of birth recently. The number of midwives declined from 75,517 in 1985 to 42,000 in 2001 despite a steadily increasing population to 13,280,200,000 (Table 8.1)

Since 2002, the title 'Midwife' disappeared from Chinese Ministry of Health annual statistics. All existing midwives were transformed either into nurses in urban areas or doctors in rural institutions. This was at the height of the implementation of the infamous 'one-child policy'.

Table 8.1 Number of midwives in China, 1949–2001

Year	1949	1957	1965	1975	1985	1990	1995	1997	1998	2001
Midwives	13,900	35,774	45,639	64,875	75,517	58,397	48,997	48,723	48,696	42,000

Source: Chinese Ministry of Health, www.moh.gov.cn/open/statistics/jb98/t2.html.

In the 2000s, while midwives were non-existent, nurses and medical staff were increasing their power within maternity care as they were perceived as symbolising science. A 100% hospital confinement rate was sought and birth became a routine event, accomplished with speed and efficiency (CMoH et al. 2003). Hospitals and their maternity care workers, thus, became the state's instrument to ensure the implementation of the one-child policy. If they failed to achieve the target set by their institutions, their salaries would be cut and their bonuses would be forfeited. One of the midwives we interviewed in this study was brave enough to report that each hospital she worked in had a small graveyard to dispose of those unplanned newborns, without parental consent. The irony of this practice is that it leads to and facilitates the survival and continuation of traditional birth attendants' (TBAs') activities of rural and urban traditions reported in Chapters 9 and 10. As a result, many midwives left midwifery, if they could make their living by other means.

'Midwife' as a symbol of a profession

The term *midwife* has its meaning in its own society, such as in China where it has been expanded to include obstetric nurses, obstetricians and doulas. Many health workers in Cheung et al.'s study (2005b) said that it did not matter what midwives were called and who did the midwifery tasks, as long as those tasks are done (see Chapter 5). We argue that this is an irresponsible fallacy that has been introduced into thinking by an abuse of power. This replicates the bitter contest between female midwives and the male-dominated medical profession in the 18th century in England (Donnison 1988), causing obstetric interventions to enter the domain of normal childbirth. Active management of birth has been used far too often to disadvantage midwives, who use their practical knowledge and manual skills to assist birth and birthing. Clearly, increasing obstetric intervention has led to the demise of Chinese midwifery. Midwifery in China has become contaminated with obstetrics now. It has no longer any specific meaning and context.

The newly acquired meanings of *Chinese midwife* are unnecessary and confusing. If the term is a symbol, it should have its meaning defined by its context. It was reported to be a symbol of backwardness in 2002 (People's Daily 2002). Now it is being changed following the struggle of Chinese midwives, the establishment of a 'midwife-led unit' and the support of the ICM (see Chapter 5). Enlightened Chinese midwives are learning from the experience and practices of other communities and communicate what they have learnt with their own communities. This symbolic meaning is implicitly an assertion that midwives are well-educated, independent, safe practitioners, who deserve respect from their communities.

The term *midwife* is culture-bound because it varies with and within the country or setting, for example, the differences between the US, the UK and Holland. Childbearing and childbirth are so culturally important that midwifery is indispensable, and no society can manage without this profession.

Discussion

Although Chinese culture is one of the earliest civilisations known, its indigenous midwifery culture has undergone changes over time. It was basically transformed into a biomedical model in the late 20th century and has been gradually disappearing since 1993, with the discontinuation of midwifery education and substitution by obstetric nurses, obstetricians and 'doulas'. The culture of the 'doula' has flourished since 1996 while 100% hospital confinement has been the aim. Simultaneously, 100% caesarean rates and midwives' redundancies are occurring. These errors have been made by health policy-makers because of lack of foresight and lack of midwifery research.

We draw the following conclusions from this: First, there is a need for midwifery services. Second, the present state of midwifery in China is a product of state policies. The state's responsibility is a commitment to ensure the quality of maternity care and to protect the interests of women. It is essential to have state legislation to support midwives' roles through a code of practice, standards, responsibilities and accountability. In this way midwifery care will become a real choice for women. Finally, more research should be commissioned by the state to investigate certain questions, which are not unique to China and apply equally to other cultures with a midwifery tradition. For example,

- Why have midwives been replaced by doctors and doulas? Is this a way to modernise maternity services?
- How can the organisation of Chinese midwifery be structured to make it a true choice for women in China?
- Can normal birth centres or home births be made possible for women in China? What are the opportunities inherent in these two types of midwifery care?
- How will Chinese women come to understand the benefits of non-interventive, midwife-supported birth?

Part III

Prospects for midwives and midwifery

In Part III, we consider the prospects for midwives and midwifery in China. In this part, drawing on interviews, historical data and literature, we illustrate the personal experience and the professional understanding of people who have been midwives in the past and/or currently. These experiences and ideas reveal more issues facing midwifery as an important part of women's health care. By relating this material to the issues addressed in Parts I and II, we conclude by considering the prospects for midwifery in China.

Our study of 'midwifery in China' would be meaningless without midwives. It is crucial for people to know something about their life, work and feelings, as they are the principal carers in the maternity services in China. If we take their entire 'subjectivities' into account, we can be more 'objective' because they, as individuals and their society, are inseparable. They are moulded by that society through their acquired skills and behaviours. Their social acquisitions are transmitted by the agency of their knowledge, the process of their learning, accumulation and assimilation of the experience and behaviour of past generations.

We study the life and work of Chinese midwives, not because of their existence but to become more aware of their importance in the care of women and newborns. Their stories in the past are intelligible to us only in the light of the present, and we can fully understand the present only in the light of the past. Midwives' past needs us to interpret and to make sense of it; without such an engagement of interpretation and reflection, the facts of what they did and experienced are unintelligible and dead. This interaction between history and facts is 'a dialogue between the historian in the present and the facts of the past' (Carr 1986: 29). This interpretive understanding involves knowing not just what the story is about but also what meaning the story actually signifies (Haralambos & Holborn 2008: 844).

Chinese midwives of the past are a social phenomenon and a fact of life. They are both the product and the conscious or unconscious orators of the society to which they belonged. It is in this capacity that their lives and work are approached here, to enable us to understand them and their professional development in order to transform and improve present-day Chinese midwifery.

9   Chinese midwives' life and
work since 770 BCE

Introduction: midwives and society

Before embarking on further exploration, we should ensure a clear understanding of why we should learn about Chinese midwives' stories.

Midwives are individuals who constitute part of society, and who are immersed in and defined by their society. Their relationships with women and society are interdependent and inseparable because, first, they contribute directly and indirectly to women's birthing experiences. Second, their clients and society would seek to avoid falling birth rates and rising mortality rates, with their implications for the population as human beings. The identification of midwives' roles provides an understanding of interaction and role theories (Turner 1991: 93, 431–4), which are relatively simple but essential.

Because society is concerned about maternity care, midwives and medical professionals have to decide what they can offer to their society in new and changing circumstances. The self-concept of individuals tends to stress the roles that are important and significant and that they can perform well. As a result, their interactive relationship with their society functions like the classic chicken-and-egg conundrum. This invites the question of which comes first: the individuals or the society (Carr 1986: 25) Both of them are necessary and complementary to each other.

Guided by the paradigm of this dialectical thinking, the relationship between a Chinese midwife and her society can be seen from an example of a child being born into this world; on one hand, her genetic make-up is complete and fixed at the moment of conception, and on the other hand, she has little control over her life. Her life is heavily shaped by the family, community and ethnic group that she is in. She has no innate choice over which language she will learn to speak. It is decided by her parents. Her acquisition of language, skills and behaviour are transmitted by the process of her learning, accumulating and assimilation of the experience and behaviour of others.

The cultural imprint as a pattern of perceptions and expectations influences the way people think and the way they express themselves, both verbally and nonverbally. The awareness of this cultural imprint can be heightened when migrating to a new culture and separation experience takes place. This challenging situation, confronted by migrants, illustrates that culture is a pattern of perceptions accepted and expected by others in a society (Nimmo 2000). The sociologist Peter Berger (1966) characterised this perspective as 'seeing the general in the particular', meaning that sociologists identify general patterns of social life in the behaviour of particular individuals.

The preceding example highlights the importance of the coherent link between a midwife and society. Therefore, it is in this capacity, that we have to learn about the lives and experiences of Chinese midwives in history and the present; thus, we will understand them, their profession and their transformation in Chinese society.

The lives of midwives have been obscured both in the past and present by the indifference of history and time. This is because of their gender and their marginal social position. In this chapter we reconstruct a picture of the life and work of Chinese midwives in history. This covers individual midwives, who were real people. Their images can be glimpsed in the archives of the period concerned. Stories of their successes, their struggles and their lives have been collected. This may involve questions of how genuine and sincere these stories are, what meaning they try to convey and in what context. The present chapter stitches together the bits and pieces of information gathered by the authors in their literature reviews and their fieldwork to portray this group of people. These experiences reveal the social construction of the lives of midwives in China; they offer insights into some ordinary, yet ambiguous, meanings that shape Chinese midwives' notions of themselves and their actions in daily life.

Artefacts

The first issue discussed here is the sources, scope and complexity of the historical account. This starts with the study of some artefacts such as carvings, a delivery kit for a birthing woman, birth certificates, and midwives' certificates.

To understand and reconstruct an image of Chinese midwives, we examined two remarkable cliff-side rock carvings identified in our fieldwork to reconstruct the birthing scene and culture in ancient China. They are the two sculptures of midwives attending births in the Southern *Sòng* dynasty (1127–1279 CE), situated in *DàZú* County, near metropolitan *Chóngqìng*, *Sìchuān* Province (see Figure 2.1, Map of China). The *Sòng* dynasty (960–1279 CE) was not as prosperous as the *Táng* dynasty (618–907 CE) had been, but scientific advances were made and great works of art and porcelain were completed. The cliff-side carving in *DàZú* was one of these amazing undertakings. A total of 50,000 statues were carved during the early *Táng* dynasty with a deliberate eye to the future. They stand there, unmoved through the centuries, proof of the skills and complexity of Chinese civilisation. Two of the sculptures (Figure 9.1) illustrate midwives' activities and many other unselfconscious areas of human life.

This outstanding sculpture reveals a birthing story from the past. The woman was giving birth in a standing position. She was supported from behind by a birth attendant, with another kneeling beside her. Both birth attendants appear to be strong and middle-aged. The main tools they used were their hands, since the care provided during childbirth was essentially based on massage, pressure and women's mobility. The gesture of the birthing woman shows that she was having labour pains. This carving illustrates how ordinary midwives worked

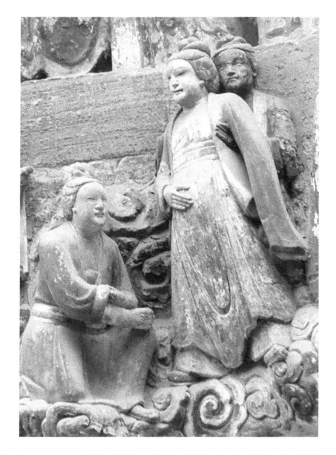

Figure 9.1 A woman was giving birth and attended by two traditional midwives.

Source: Photograph by the authors, 2008.

Notes: The statue was carved in *Sòng* dynasty between 1127 and 1279 CE. It is one of the *DàZú* cliff-side rock carvings in the west of *Chóngqìng* City.

and how women gave birth during the *Sòng* dynasty. The birthing position the woman adopts shows the impossibility of modern midwifery and obstetric manoeuvres, such as guarding the perineum and episiotomy. The carving also shows the watchfulness of the midwives and their readiness to assist the baby's birth. These records of birthing and midwifery stories pre-dated by centuries those in Germany, France, Spain, Italy and the UK (Donnison 1988; Towler & Bramall 1986; Ortiz 1993; Gelbart 1993a, b; Marland 1993; Tew 1998).

To shed further light on the features of a midwife at that time and in particular her social position, we observe another caving showing a birthing woman in an upright sitting position with her midwife nearby (Figure 9.2a). The caving is situated in the lowest realm of hell in the configuration of a Buddhist 'Wheel of Life' (Figure 9.2b) which was carved between 1174 and 1252.

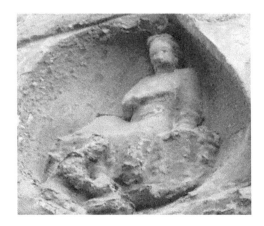

Figure 9.2a Giving birth in a sitting upright position in the Southern Song dynasty

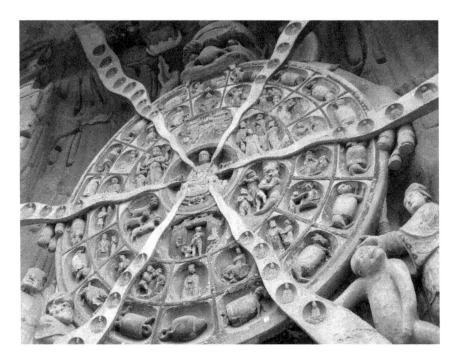

Figure 9.2b Buddhist Wheel of Life (carved between 1174 and 1252)
Source: Photograph by the authors, 2008.

The Wheel of Life is 780 cm high, 480 cm wide and 260 cm deep. It shows the Buddhist concept of the six realms of existence into which humans can be reborn. No clear interpretation has been provided for this huge wheel on the site of *DàZú* in south-west China. We can find that this wheel has been presented in a different way from other presentations throughout the Buddhist world, for example, a Tibetan one. According to the Tibetan Buddhist interpretation, the six realms are the realms of (1) the gods (top centre), (2) the Titans (demigods; top left), (3) the humans (top right), (4) the animals (bottom left), (5) the hungry ghosts (bottom right) and (6) hell (bottom centre; Thurman 2006). The wheel houses 90 statues of people and 24 statues of animals. The rebirth into the next life rests on the behaviours in one's past life. To break free of the cycle good deeds are necessary while still alive.

Being depicted in the realm of hell tells us something of the social attitude towards childbirth at that time. It might have conveyed an idea that childbirth involves suffering and hardship. This shows a negative image of women in labour, a life event which in fact has been so important to many. A birth attendant (the midwife) has been shown alongside with this woman in labour, which might have served as an indicator of birthing but which nevertheless carries a negative impact for the occupation. The image of the suffering in labour has gone so far as to consort with the devil. So, the interpretations we can come to are, first, giving birth is perceived as painful, being a form of torture; second, attending birth is not an admirable job.

These two carvings reveal clearly that throughout recorded history childbearing women have been assisted by other women. Birth attendants formed one of the ancient female occupations in China and elsewhere (Marland 1993; Donnison 1988). The carvings also show us two widely used birthing positions of the time (standing and sitting) which might have been forgotten in China nowadays. This historical evidence challenges the recumbent birthing positions developed in the 18th and 19th centuries

They support further that many stereotypes of features of traditional midwives developed as time went by, for instance, weak in nature but strong in health and domestic care (Lee 2003, 2008). They were old, warm-hearted and less educated or ignorant. However, they assumed unique caring roles in women's growing families, regardless of demands on their own time and sometimes their health, resulting from multiple caring roles.

Chinese midwives' gender and society

It is difficult to go far into discussion of the experiences and social relationships between midwives and society without encountering their gender and social position. The first social and political issue confronting Chinese midwives in history and currently is their gender. Chinese midwifery was respectable before the *Sòng* dynasty and gradually lost its original position as schools were closed to females (Leung 2000: 105–10). Apart from attending births, suspicion was aggravated by their role relating to the female sexual body, such as in legal cases to check young women's virginity, to examine the quality of wet nurses' milk in the imperial palace and to check corpses to assess whether sexual assault or pregnancy was involved. Midwives became less respectable by the time of the *Míng* dynasty (1368–1644), especially when occupations were classified as *sāngūliùpó* ('the three aunties and six grannies'; Guide – Chinese glossary).

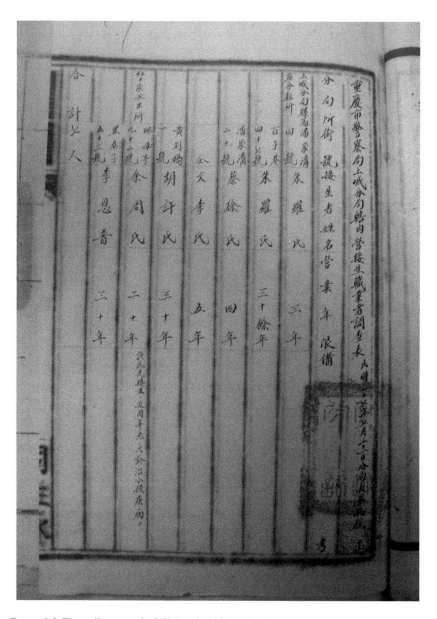

Figure 9.3 The police record of *Chóngqìng* birth attendants

Source: *Chóngqìng* National Archives; photograph by the authors, 2008.

The occupation of midwifery became the lowest of all walks of life (Leung 2000: 102).

Midwives constant involvement in childbirth, birthing blood, body fluids and female sexual bodies gave them a certain power. This not only was because children would carry on family names but also made midwives susceptible to accusations of carrying pollution as social beings (Ahern 1978c; Leung 2000: 111). However, despite these negative aspects of their image, they remained unchallenged in the care of childbirth in Chinese history (Leung 2000: 112). Midwifery developed as an occupation in pre-modern China, then a profession in modern China and gradually deteriorated to mingle with nursing and medicine and then struggle to be a semi-profession presently.

Because China is a male-dominated society, the gender of midwives and social constructs threaten them with marginalisation. This can be observed from a page (Figure 9.3) of the registration list recorded by *Chóngqìng* Municipal Police Department in 1938.

This page of a survey investigation records seven birth attendants/midwives living under the catchment areas in the Upper City Branch of *Chóngqìng* Police Station, which will be further discussed in later in this chapter. Six of them did not have their own names, but their husband's surname plus the surnames of the woman's family. Although they had been in business supporting women and their family for either more than 3 or to 30 years, they were nobody but subordinate to their and their spouse's families.

As a result, their lives and work have received little attention, and their profession is presently in decline because of medicalisation of childbirth, industrialisation of the country and transformation of attitudes toward hospital delivery (CMoH et al. 2003; Cheung 2009). Chinese midwives, however, are still playing a role in intrapartum care but have become less important.

Social stratification

The ranking of midwives in their communities was determined by their position in the social hierarchy or, in other words, their income, wealth, power, age and status (Barnard & Spencer 2002: 623). This approach can be considered as a system of structured inequalities that persist over time.

Traditional Chinese midwives came from various strata in society, where there were always two groups of them: the wealthier and the poorer. They, like today, were mainly from working-class families. Most of their families could not afford to have their daughters' feet bound (Hays 2013), as their families needed helping hands within and outside the house. This was especially true in southern China, as peasants had to grow two or three crops of rice a year. Chinese midwives were relatively isolated from the population by their occupation, which was closely related to their lower social status and their economic deprivation. However, they had to be responsible for both their clients and their own families. The more experienced midwives were appointed by local authorities to the court to serve the emperor's family, while the rest continued serving their communities.

China is a huge country where the differences between the lives of the rich and the poor are very great. Advances in science and technology during the early 20th century greatly changed the lives of people in China and around the world. The lives of the modern-day Chinese midwives are no exception, especially since 1928.

The head of the first Chinese state midwifery school

Yáng Chóngruì (杨崇瑞; see Chapter 4) was born in 1891 in a village in *Tōng* County, *Héběi* Province, and died in 1983. She was trained as an obstetrician in the missionary Peking Union Medical College (PUMC) and did her postgraduate study in the Public Health Department at the Johns Hopkins Medical College in Baltimore.

When she returned from America, she was sufficiently enlightened to recognise the high maternal and neonatal mortality resulting from tetanus. This was because traditional midwives had poor hygiene and no knowledge of or skills in asepsis. Armed with the Chinese Ministry of Health's (CMoH'S) Midwives Rules and the Traditional Birth Attendant Management Rules from the Ministry of the Interior (see Chapter 4), she helped to establish the first *Běipíng* Birth Attendant School in 1928 (see Chapter 3) and then the first state-approved midwifery school in *Qílín Hútòng Běijīng* in 1929 (see Chapter 3; MCHDMH 1991; *Yáng & Wáng* 2007). She became head of both schools, promoting midwifery care and family planning, but she did not abandon Chinese traditional birth attendants, regarding them as re-trainable in modern midwifery. Since then, Chinese midwifery rose, for the first time, to become a profession.

Although she did not seek to improve Chinese midwifery after the communist government came to power in 1949, she quickly became famous for her work in maternity care after her death. The centenary of her birth was celebrated by the Department of Maternity-Child Health, the Chinese Ministry of Health in 1991.

Birth attendants

Using the literature review and other material available, we are looking at Chinese birth attendants in the two cities of *Chóngqìng* and *Guǎngzhōu*.

Chóngqìng

Chóngqìng in south-west China became the capital on 1 December 1937 during the Sino-Japanese War after the central government retreated there. There was an attempt in the subsequent year to provide birth attendants with basic midwifery training, facilitated by a police survey recording their names, home addresses and length of practice in the city see the above Figure 9.3.

A total of 28 TBAs in *Chóngqìng* were recorded in the document. The average experience as a TBA was over 21 years, with many having been in the job for all of their working lives. The local government attempted to transform them into biomedical-trained birth attendants, but there is no evidence of success.

Guăngzhōu

Some stories of the birth attendants in *Guăngzhōu* city, *Guăngdōng Province,* China (see Figure 2.1) were reported in the *Southern Daily* (Ma & Cheng 2006). The TBAs attracted business through a wooden sign hanging on the front door of their house in the 1940s and 1950s. on the sign was printed: 'Aunty . . . birth attendance and housekeeping' (*mŏushì shōuxĭ*; Guide – Chinese glossary). They attracted business through their network of friends and relatives. Many of them did not charge for their services but expected a gift in return.

Family life at that time was close and families were large. Women clung to the traditions of their mothers, and the majority of babies were born at home – by gasoline light. Water often had to be carried in a pair of wooden buckets with a shoulder-pole and boiled up in an iron pot for the traditional birth attendant. People chose TBAs because they did not like to have their baby in hospital with male medical staff present (Ma & Cheng 2006). Therefore, the development of a biomedical model of midwifery was not straightforward.

The life of a birth attendant was much the same everywhere. She was just one of those ordinary housewives. She was a tie that helped keep the community in harmony. This harmony allowed the family to expand without undue disruption. She was always received with respect, being considered a learned and experienced woman.

Birth attendants based their practice on careful observation and their personal experience of childbirth, including symptoms and effects of any intervention. Being illiterate, they passed on their knowledge and skills orally. This way of transferring their knowledge reflected their low social status, meaning that throughout history they have found it difficult to earn a living.

A legal framework for midwives

Midwives in China had been subjected to governmental regulations and laws one way or another since 1913 (see Chapter 4), at least wherever governmental bodies had the administrative means to do so. Before that we have been unable to locate any governmental documents indicating concern with midwifery practice, even throughout the Chinese empires or dynasties. It may be said that, alongside the paradigmatic shift in Chinese medical practices (i.e. becoming Europeanised), the governmental regulations and laws marked the beginning of the modernisation of midwifery practice in China. What we need to understand now, is how far and in what way regulations and laws modernised Chinese midwifery practice.

In 1928, the first Biomedical Midwives Rules were issued by the Chinese Ministry of Health and the codes of conduct were revised once in 1929. It was not

until 1943 that the Midwifery Laws were issued by the central Chinese Nationalist Government (1943), but these laws were also the last ones in mainland China
from then on, due to the turmoil of wars and revolutions. In the meantime, before
1949, we found provincial governments designing and revising rules based on
central government rules for midwifery education and practice. For example, in
1936, the *Sìchuān* provincial government in south-west China issued an order to
its capital city council stating that the 1929 central government examination system had been revised and that the new rules would be implemented immediately
(see Figure 9.4 showing the original copy of the order).

The change of government in 1949 in mainland China may have been a reason for the discontinuation of central Nationalists' governmental regulations and
laws for midwifery practice, in association with greater political centralisation.
It is also notable that in the next three decades no specific regulations were produced concerning midwifery, birth or birthing care. In our research, not even
regulations relating to medical care were found! Ironically, these periods were
the golden times of a 'baby boom' in mainland China. Despite a period of famine

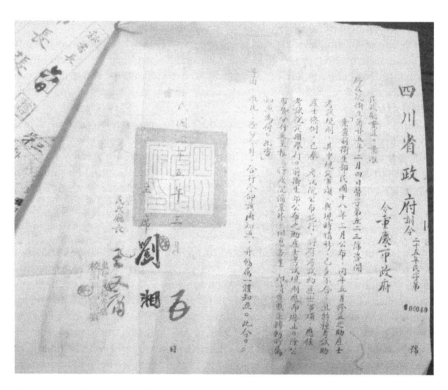

Figure 9.4 A *Sìchuān* provincial government document to abolish the old examination
rules for midwives

Source: *Chóngqìng* National Archives 0053–24–68; photograph by the authors, 2008.

(1959–1961) and a period of further political turmoil akin to a civil war, which claimed many lives (1966–1969), the population of mainland China continued to grow. We can imagine that in these periods, so far as birthing care and births were concerned, traditional midwives in different regions of China played important roles, especially in rural areas, even though they were almost unregulated and had little organised training. The 1943 central government's regulations were no longer implemented after 1949 and were quickly abandoned because of the change of government. Such rationales as had been produced in these regulations for midwifery practice, nevertheless, could have been used in state hospitals under the new government.

So far as health care was concerned, the two modern Chinese governments, the one in Taiwan and the other on the mainland, did have something in common. Health services, including birthing care, were only funded for employees of government departments, organisations and enterprises, which were only about 10% of the population. The rest of the population either had to pay or buy their insurance for treatments and services in state hospitals or consult self-employed practitioners trained in Chinese or European medicine. These arrangements applied equally to women seeking maternity care, by either state hospital-employed midwives trained by modern midwifery schools, or self-employed midwives, usually traditional birth attendants.

In the 1960s, the government organised some health services for the, mainly rural, population of 630 million people at that time (1960–1970). In 1968 the system of so-called barefoot doctors was created. It was a kind of cooperative medical insurance in which villagers or people in the private sectors paid a small premium for health care provided by 'barefoot doctors'.

'Barefoot' implied that the doctor was a peasant working part-time in the fields and providing health services part-time. Some also became full-time doctors. Midwifery either became part of the female barefoot doctors' job or continued to be performed by village granny midwives. The 'barefoot doctor' practice did not include a systematic maternity care arrangement.

'Barefoot doctoring' shifted care away from state hospitals to urban and rural clinics. It did ease the workload of the limited state hospitals and helped increase medical coverage, at least in structural terms. This system was known in China as a 'co-operative health care service', alongside the limited 'state health care service'. Most 'barefoot doctors', whose duty, apart from that of a doctor, would include those of nurses, midwives (if they were female), dentists and other medical auxiliaries; they were recruited from the private traditional Chinese medicine-men or some traditional midwives who otherwise had some Chinese medical knowledge. Their biomedical knowledge was limited because of being self-taught. The Chinese government nevertheless provided brief training (ranging from one to six months) to selected barefoot doctors in hospitals, state medical colleges or universities. Still, outside both the state healthcare service and the 'barefoot doctor' co-operative service, the private traditional Chinese midwives or birth attendants were functioning (see Chapter 10).

In southern China in the 1970s, the estimated ratio of traditional midwives to total population was about 1:600. The figure may appear reasonable, but the services were not. Most of them were part-time untrained people, as observed by one of our authors (NFC) when she was recruited as a 'barefoot doctor' in the early 1970s in southern China.

The barefoot doctor scheme was a cooperative system to tackle the acute shortage of medicine and doctors during the Cultural Revolution in China's urban and, especially, rural communities in the late 1960s and 1970s. It was the government's strategy to shift the health care burden to the communities. Most barefoot doctors, especially the older ones, had no formal training, but some younger ones had three, six or twelve months training before practising medicine. Their jobs involved providing primary health care for, for example, minor illnesses, immunisations, education, maternal and child health care. The quality of their care was, of course, very basic. However, this experience, in some way, inspired the World Health Organization to launch the Health for All by 2000 programme.

The problem with 'barefoot doctors' who acted as midwives was that they often had inadequate training and preparation to carry out antenatal, intrapartum and postnatal care in clinics and mothers' homes. They sometimes encountered complications, particularly, malpresentation, obstruction of labour and postpartum haemorrhage. Without proper medical back-up, they risked endangering the health of women and their newborns. It was such questionable practices that led to the unjustifiable conclusions and regulations stipulated in a government health report (CMoH et al. 2003). All mothers were required to deliver in large hospitals, home birth was to be phased out and the midwife's role was to be reduced to that of obstetricians' handmaidens. The conclusion of the report failed to see that place of birth was not the only issue to ensure the safety of mothers and their newborns, but midwifery education, support for midwives and proper regulation of their conduct were and are crucial.

The registration of college-trained midwives has been deleted from the statistics registry of the Ministry of Health in China since 2001. All midwives have had to register and be counted as either nurses or doctors in the government's statistics and their employment. This brought about the official disappearance of midwives in maternity services, though staff working in the birthing room still call themselves and are known as midwives.

On the basis of this brief review of the regulations for midwives we would argue that statutory regulations and midwives' education should be founded on research evidence. Midwives should regain their status and responsibility in the care of healthy childbearing women and assume control of midwifery education. If midwives are not in control of their education, inappropriate decisions and policies concerning students' clinical learning experiences could impair their developing skills.

A small group of highly educated and vocal midwives are able to form a pressure group for the advancement of their calling (Cheung et al. 2005a, b, 2006a, b; Mander & Cheung 2006; Cheung 2009). The leaders of this new group would play, in the coming decade, a vital part in the battle for the reinstatement of midwifery as a respectable profession in China.

A nurse-midwife in *Níngxià*

The need for change is highlighted by the experience of a nurse midwife aged 104, *Shìjié Chéng*, which was reported in 2006 from *Yínchuān*, the capital of *Níngxià Huí* Autonomous Region (*Níngxià* Daily 2006). She was trained as a nurse in *Pǔài* Nursing School of a missionary hospital, in *Hànkǒu*, in central China. After her studies she went to work in *Yínchuān* in 1934 with three of her colleagues, offering their services free to the local communities, but in return they faced hostility. The local residents shut doors in their faces, let dogs attack them or used a broom to show them the door. Local people continued to use traditional birth attendants, who tied the childbearing woman's hair to the beam of the house to keep her chin up during labour. The baby was born onto a layer of yellow sand prepared beforehand. Ms *Chéng*'s colleagues found difficulty coping and left, but she stayed on. It took her years of perseverance to convince local people that asepsis at the birth was good for the health of babies and mothers. On this micro-level action approach, we can see that her activity helped to make her, and her profession, visible locally and nationally.

To look at this story from another level, we can sense that the Chinese midwifery reported focuses mainly on labour. It is likely that there was no antenatal care, and there was nobody involved until labour started. Midwifery, though, should not be seen just in term of labour or birthing. This is not the midwife's role and never was, even before pre-modern times. For centuries, Chinese midwives' focus has been on the rights of women, and midwives have made important contributions to women's health (*Fù* 1425).

Midwives in the 21st century are still conditioned and constrained by their fellow health workers and their social environment, making the profession the product of the society. The understanding of the development of the profession has been built on medical assumptions. Chinese midwives have been created by a system they could not alter. Should they seek to change their professional practice and standards, informed by their past and those in the other parts of the world? This is a difficult question which appears to be impossible for Chinese midwives alone to answer since much of the decision-making is in the hands of politicians or their medical colleagues. Unfortunately, this historical evidence has demonstrated the complexities of the social and professional quandary in which Chinese midwives find themselves.

Discussion

In this chapter we have addressed three points. First, Chinese midwifery history encompasses diverse sources and scope, for example, artefacts, gender issues, their social position, stratification and so on. Second is the development of Chinese midwifery, which takes many forms: significant individuals, midwifery associations and societies. Third, the development of midwifery regulations and Chinese midwifery's somewhat marginal position compared to nursing and medicine.

Our study of the lives and experience of Chinese midwives in written materials has provided windows onto the past. It has highlighted how midwifery and its education perpetuate professional inequality. The lives of Chinese midwives in the past can only be intelligible to us in the light of the present, and their present can only be fully understood in the light of the past. Their lives and work are both the product and the conscious or unconscious orators of the society to which they belong. Their past needs us to interpret and to make sense; without such an engagement of understanding, interpretation and reflection, the facts of what they did and experienced are unintelligible and dead.

10 Modern midwives' stories (1929–2017 CE)

Introduction

Chinese midwives should be understood through, not only an understanding of their past but also of their present situation in modern China. The stories of the midwives we interviewed in China will improve understanding of their views and perspectives. They are the primary sources by which we can judge the reliability of the historical knowledge of Chinese midwifery. This approach also incorporates the study of a wide range of other primary materials and the evaluation of a range of accounts to inform us of what has happened in Chinese midwifery.

In this investigation, we carried out field research and interviews with 38 people from five villages, 12 cities and four municipalities across 13 provinces in China. Among them six were birth attendants, 20 nurse-midwives/midwives and 12 midwifery leaders and academics.

Little is known about the lives and work of Chinese midwives in history and even less has been written about them recently. These people, whose services relate to everybody in China, do not deserve to be marginalised. The absence of an account of their work would be a source of regret for maternity care in modern China and for midwives worldwide.

First of all, we shall relate the experience of one of the authors as a midwife in southern China and the UK. She might have a unique experience as an individual practitioner, but her career facilitates understanding of midwifery services in the 21st century, when China was still undergoing turbulent struggles on its way to modernise. The experience of both authors as midwives and researchers facilitate our understanding of the lives and experiences of those midwives interviewed, against the background presented in Chapters 3 and 4. It is widely accepted that healthcare is a political issue in modern nation states. In view of the advances in science and technology, this applies to maternity as much as to any other aspect of health. We have two reasons for saying this: one was the uncertainty concerning midwifery education in China in the past decades, as discussed in Chapter 4. Another is the existence of a range of agencies providing birthing care in modern China, as will be seen in our stories of modern Chinese midwives. In other words, midwifery services have not previously been seriously considered in either theory or practice or the structure of health care provision in China.

Modern midwives' stories

Some of the names used in these stories are real and some are pseudonyms, as preferred by the participants. We came to know them through friends and our social networks.

An urban traditional midwife

Ms *Yáng Shūfāng* (Figure 10.1a) in *Hándān* City, *Héběi* Province, was introduced to us by a local hospital midwifery manager in 2008. The city has a recorded history of more than 3,000 years and a population of more than 9,433 million in 2015 (*Hándān* Statistic Bureau 2016). When we arrived at her clinic (Figure 10.1b) after a 36-hour train journey, she was having a consultation session in her clinic in a high street near a farmers' market. The woman client was pregnant for the second time,

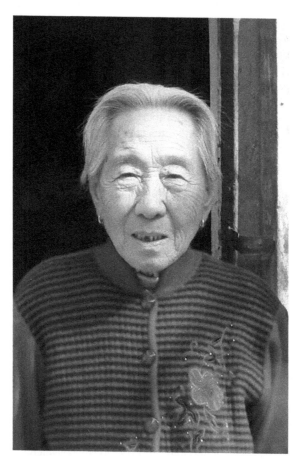

Figure 10.1a Ms *Yáng*
Source: Photograph by the authors.

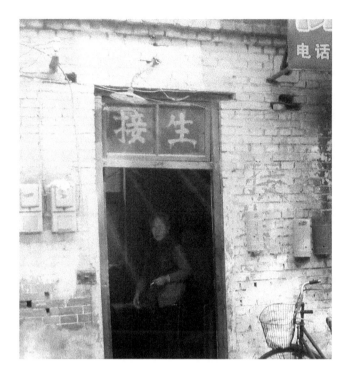

Figure 10.1b Ms *Yáng*'s birthing centre in *Hándān* City, *Héběi* Province
Source: Photograph by the authors.

and her mother was present. Ms *Yáng* was, like thousands of other traditional mid-wives, working quietly in her community where people were born, lived and died.

Ms *Yáng* was already 87 years old, but she was quite witty and fit for her age. She had an unusually high and healthy self-esteem, though she was unable to read or write. She told us with pride that she had attended births for 55 years with no foetal or maternal deaths. She had neither attended any school nor listened to any lecturers on female anatomy. She had learned her trade through word of mouth, hands-on experience and a period of informal apprenticeship with an elderly lady doctor. Her knowledge also included material gleaned from her husband, who was trained as a doctor in the army. This could be observed from the birthing kit she used, which was similar to those in any village clinic (Figure 10.1c). There were cotton wool balls, two pairs of stainless steel artery forceps and a pair of stainless steel scissors for cutting the cord. She sterilised the kit with steam and cleaned the woman's skin with alcohol – a practice uncommon among traditional midwives and birth attendants in China.

She had operated her three-room birth centre for many years with some support from family members who worked in local hospitals and health authority departments. She had contrasting qualities: illiterate and untidy in her workplace

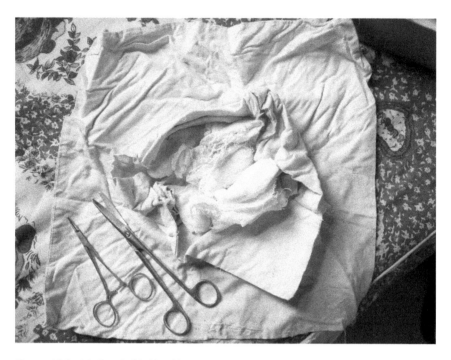

Figure 10.1c Ms *Yáng*'s birthing kit
Source: Photograph by the authors.

but kind-hearted and keen to learn. The wooden birthing bed she used in the birth centre was designed by her and made by a carpenter. Innovatively, the bed had a handle on each side for the woman to hold when pushing to give birth. She showed us around her clinic and her equipment with obvious pride. It is amazing that her birth centre had survived up to this time, when no one was allowed to practise without a relevant qualification and a licence, especially in the centre of the city.

The good thing for Ms *Yáng* in her urban area as a traditional midwife was that she could practise regularly, especially in the period when the state-controlled health care provision came to a halt or became dysfunctional, as happened in the 1966–1976 Cultural Revolution. Local people used her birth centre quite a lot at that time because many hospitals were closed. Attending both normal and complicated births, she served city officials as well as the poor, helping several generations of the same families. She soon became well known to many households for her work and her kindness.

The birth centre was able to provide basic maternity services at people's convenience, and she attended home births, saying:

> When I was pregnant with my youngest daughter, I was fetched to attend a home birth. Normally a pregnant woman would not be allowed to attend

childbirth, but I did. I had to do it because the family needed me. If I did not do it, they could not find anyone.

She was right that she was badly needed at that time when the system was too narrowly based, too feeble and too corrupt to solve the problems which faced communities. Since then Ms *Yáng*'s reputation grew, and people continued to use her services. Even when she grew old and could not attend births, people still came to seek her advice and stay at her house prior to admission to hospital. She could still make some referrals and sometimes escorted her client to the hospital:

> When she started to have regular contractions, she came to me. I did a check for her. Her cervix is only a figure tip. I told her it was too early to go into hospital. She stayed with me for about four to five hours. I did another examination for her and found that her cervix was nearly fully dilated. I then prompted her to go to hospital. When the hospital staff did the exam, they discovered it was too late for a [caesarean] section now. I told them that if you want to give birth yourself, don't go to hospital too early.

When transferring a woman, the maternity hospital would pay her from 100 to 200 yuan (£10–20) 'introductory fee'. The fee paid by the hospital implied their recognition of her referral. How exactly this arrangement and amount came about we do not know. However, she is typical of midwifery in her society, and her experiences tell the inside story of maternity practice in this part of China.

What made her service so special? She told us that during labour, she stayed with the woman throughout. She tried hard to encourage the woman to give birth naturally. In addition, she made her services available 24 hours a day and seven days a week and would refer women to maternity hospitals if necessary. She had developed a deep commitment, as well as a gratitude to women. They were loyal to her for good reasons: especially the skilful and individualised care that she could provide locally. Her reward was continuing opportunities to practise, to learn and to make her living as a traditional midwife.

According to her, she never did, in her working life, an episiotomy, induction or augmentation of labour, and there were no serious tears or deaths in her care. If there were any haemorrhages or tears, she would use two forceps to clamp the bleeding spot to stop bleeding; alternatively, she would clamp the tear to facilitate its eventual closure and healing. In the last decade, as caesarean almost became a fashionable way of giving birth in maternity hospitals in China, if women chose to give birth naturally, they would employ her, with advice to delay admission, to avoid caesarean. Her tales reflected her adjustment and resistance to the new and competing roles of the medical mainstream. She was neither patronising nor undermining of women's agency in her counselling, which is a laudable and a unique example of 'being with' women. This was not atypical, as all traditional birth attendants/midwives we interviewed practised similarly.

The fact remained that her practice was unlicenced, despite regulations in China that no unqualified people can operate a birthing room, not to mention a birth centre. It looks like what we saw here was a *de facto* qualification readily accepted by birthing women, but not recognised by the state healthcare authorities. It was a situation that the health care authorities did not know what to do with or even care about. The licensing law was obviously not imposed in this case, but the public seemed unconcerned. As for Ms *Yáng*, her personal relations in the local community must have been very important for her to continue practising.

The statutory regulations and standards in maternity care are a political way of maintaining professional order and safe childbirth. But in reality, reassurance may appear in another face. Ms *Yáng's* practice did not pose any dangers or, at least, there have been no formal complaints about her. Hers was in itself a face of reassurance: her skill, her reputation in birthing care and her social relations in the community. Ms *Yáng* might have applied for a licence, but she could not because of her background. We can see that in fact both effective regulations and Ms *Yáng*'s skills are needed to reassure the public about childbirth. Suppose we have a nurse/nurse-midwife who works in a licenced maternity hospital, but who lacks the interpersonal skills possessed by Ms *Yáng*: she would not be reassuring the birthing women in her care. It seems that we have a situation here in the maternity care in this part of China where the political means to maintain care and the quality to provide care are strangers to each other. We can argue that such a dislocation of maternity care provision is a direct consequence of putting midwifery practice in a dubious position in China. If we look at the regulations about maternity care regarding midwives in China, our research into what is published shows their pathological orientation. This orientation contradicts any midwifery theory. Otherwise, Ms *Yáng* could have been licenced. The Chinese health authorities are facing a legacy of traditional talent in maternity care in China. They have to rethink the means by which care provision is ordered. Such a means has to be a complete integration of policies and practices. The disintegration of both results in talent being outlawed while lawful practices become problematic.

From the experience of Ms *Yáng*, we learn that traditional midwives were far from as ignorant as they are perceived through the eyes of technological obstetrics. They are still a part of the maternity care workforce, attend births and are birth companions in many families' lives. Their experiences demonstrate issues of gender, health policy and political economy.

Two village birth attendants

Ms Zhào Xiùlán (Figure 10.2a)

Ms *Zhào* was introduced to us by the mother of a student and was interviewed in 2013, because she was held in such high esteem by local birthing women and their families.

This 72-year-old lady greeted us at her front door and led us to her *kàng* (炕; Guide – Chinese glossary), which is the local custom during winter (Figure 10.2b). Although retired from attending births since 1990, she still has vivid memories of her training and subsequent practice in her village. She stressed that

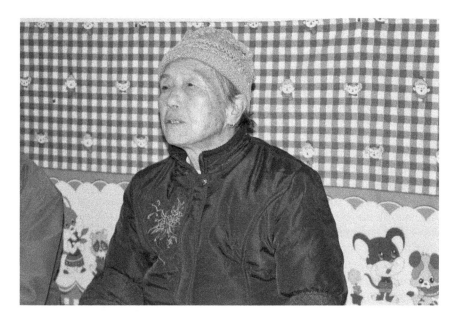

Figure 10.2a Birth attendant *Zhào Xiùlán*

Source: Photograph by the authors' assistant.

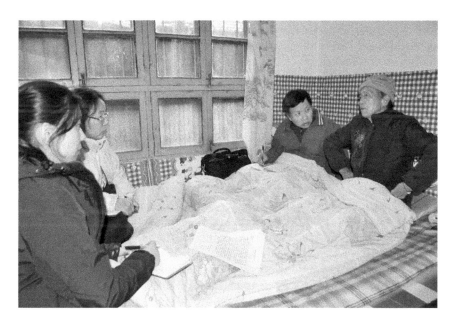

Figure 10.2b The interview took place on *Kang* at Ms *Zhào Xiùlán*'s home in November 2013

Source: Photograph by the authors' assistant.

her skills and knowledge achieved through the training from a hospital near *Xīān* in the 1950s were essential for her practice. She also stressed that her training and experience have granted her a kind of occupational status and economic security in the village. Though her service was free to women and their families, she and her family were supported by the community in return for her services.

The first 'baby' whose birth she attended is now over 45, and the last one is 14 years old. She had attended more than 1,000 births but, unfortunately, was forced to stop practising because the babies she delivered could not be registered after 2008, as she was a birth attendant. Now if she wanted, she could attend only those births where the families did not have a birth permit or those who did not care whether the birth could be registered or not.

Here we may need some background explanation to help readers understand the notion of 'birth permit' and the significance of getting the child's birth registered. In China every pregnant woman is required to obtain a birth permit to give birth from the administration office of her *hukou* (a form of household registration in the Chinese government system); and the permit needs to be issued before conception or during pregnancy to the applicant in person in the place where the household is registered. This means that the applicants have to go back to the place where their *hukou* was registered with the local National Population and Family Planning Commission (NPFPC). The enforcement of this policy creates many difficulties, particularly for those people moving around the country and prevents them from using the maternity services appropriately, thus intruding on their rights. Those who fail to obtain a birth permit risk their pregnancy and birth being considered 'unauthorised'. This causes difficulty in accessing appropriate maternity care and maternity leave, being penalised for the unauthorised birth, non-reimbursement of maternity costs, difficulty registering the birth and difficulty arranging the child's nursery care, schooling and future social benefits.

To come back to Ms *Zhào*, she emphasised once again that '[b]irth attendance needs experience':

> I normally visit the woman at their home when she is six or seven months gestation. When she is in labour, I would go and stay with her. When her cervix is 3cm dilated, I'd advise her to walk about in the house or garden. If the woman complains about the contraction pain, that is fine. If she screams and shouts 'I don't want to live', that is the sign of full dilatation of the cervix.
>
> I would ask her to semi-sitting on her bed supported by her husband and her mother on each side during the pushing phase. . . .
>
> I normally stay with the woman postnatally for more than an hour. If everything is OK I would leave her after giving her some sugary drinks and teaching her how to look after her newborn and helping her with her first time breast feeding. I'd pay return visits on postnatal day 3 and 5. If neonatal jaundice persists, I'd advised the family to take the baby to hospital. There is no need on most occasions.

Maintaining personal hygiene was also considered by her a priority. If any sign of difficult labour was predicted, she would arrange a transfer to hospital.

Ms Wàn Sùzhēn

Ms *Wàn Sùzhēn* was a village birth attendant in *Héběi* Province for more than 30 years until 2000. She enjoyed considerable personal rapport.

Ms *Wàn* learnt her midwifery skills from her experience of giving birth to her eldest son in 1963. She had a postpartum haemorrhage and stayed in hospital for about two months. It was then that a doctor persuaded her to learn some birth attending skills. On her return home, the traditional midwife in the village was old and retired. Ms *Wàn* took up the job with what she had learnt. She continued to learn by doing the job. While she was carrying out the duties of a village midwife, like other women, she bore children of her own and looked after her own family. She was able to combine these activities and was soon accepted by the local people. What she had learnt in the hospital, while she was a patient there, was a worthwhile investment.

Ms *Wàn*, like her fellow women villagers, performed all types of farm labour and household work. She faced more hardship when she had subsequent children. She had little time for herself or for leisure, but her job as a village midwife brought her extra income. Normally she was called to her client's home when the woman's family considered labour to be well established, suggesting that antenatal care was by somebody else, most likely the woman's kin or neighbours. She always kept her promise to come to help a birthing woman. She would stay with the woman until the birth was completed. This could be a day or two or even longer. After the birth, she would wash and dress the baby. She provided services not only for her village but also for neighbouring villages. Many families used her services several times. The majority of her clients expressed a high level of confidence in her skills by summoning her repeatedly for their subsequent births or by recommending her services to other family members. When there was a person who was ill, weak or had died, Ms *Wàn* also tried to help out.

Although she did not charge for her services to needy families, many of them chose to pay her out of gratitude, according to their means. The size of payment could be two to five yuans (a hospital midwife at that time earned 40 to 50 yuans per month, the sterling (British Pound, GBP) exchange rate then was £1 = 15 yuans). She was also paid in kind, with eggs, chicken, grain or pieces of cloth. Alternatively, there could be generous gifts during festivals, depending on the complexity of the delivery and quality of the care received. Generally, she was paid more by better-off families. Her service to wealthier families often became a way to show her personal fame and prestige, making her services different from those of the other birth attendants in the area. She was a respected figure in her neighbourhood. Everybody knew her and her house. Women continued to use her services throughout their childbearing years. She knew everybody in the villages in the area, being either an acquaintance or a friend of her clients.

The local government provided training in local hospitals for birth attendants like her in the 1970s and 1980s. She also received training in contraception. She was given a 'delivery kit', intra-uterine contraceptive devices (IUCDs), an insertion kit and an IUCD removal kit. She learned to use oxytocin by intra-muscular injection to speed up labour and to perform basic cardiopulmonary resuscitation.

Many women turned to her for information and intervention, but she did not approve of contraception or abortion. She stated her objection to abortion and thought this practice was wrong.

When an apnoeic baby was born, Ms *Wàn* would hold it by its feet and give it a few gentle slaps. If this did not work, she would fold the baby's head towards its knees. Usually this would do the trick. Then she would concentrate on the new mother. If the placenta was slow to deliver, she might massage her belly. She pressed the woman's belly and told her to bear down. There is not much indication from Ms *Wàn*'s story that discussion took place between the labouring woman and her about the labour progress and intervention. She gave us the impression that she was in charge at births, and she knew all there was to know about family secrets. According to her, no one died under her care in her lifetime's work. She attended such a large number of births each year that she lost count of how many. She often had to travel long distances. Her social status and her part in the life of the community made her an important person in the village.

Ms *Wàn* saw that women were able to give birth to their babies themselves; they did not need caesareans or medical treatment to give birth because those treatments or operations undermined women's constitution or strength. She blamed high caesarean rates on hospitals' greed for profit. According to her, in order to generate profits, hospitals misled women into accepting caesareans. She felt sorry that women agreed to accept the operation because of the misleading doctors. Ms *Wan* observed that in China today, lack of money denies decent health care to many, including even the relatively wealthy.

A trained birth attendant and self-taught obstetrician

Born to a peasant family in 1934 in a village in *Jiāngsū* Province, eastern China, Ms *Táo Jìngxiù* lost her father at the age of two because of the Sino-Japanese War. At the age of 15, she was lucky enough and privileged to enter a Health Experimental School in *Tōng* County, a suburb of *Běijīng*, to be trained as a labour ward birth attendant. It helped that her cousin was the general secretary of the State Council of China; her sister-in-law was then head of the Obstetric Department, Ministry of Health, and the dean of the Research Institute of Chinese Medicine. Neighbours and personal ties also helped her enter midwifery and affected the way she practised.

At the very beginning, Ms *Táo* found it difficult to accept the idea of being trained to be a birth attendant. Her mother was reluctant to let people know that her daughter was learning this. She thought there was no need for her to learn the practice of midwifery because giving birth was a job that every woman knew. She disagreed with her mother and they became estranged. Established in 1947, the school offered a crash course because of the acute shortage of trained health workers. It was designed to last for only one year and was run by an old Red Army officer, *Zhào Shìkūn*. Ms *Táo* learnt midwifery and medical technology enthusiastically, but little information was readily accessible and comprehensible to her. There were no proper textbooks, only some leaflets, which, in comparison with modern midwifery or obstetric textbooks, contained simple reproductive anatomy and simple birthing techniques. The complex moral, social and technical problems in maternity care were missing from the teaching materials of her day.

After training, Ms *Tao* was assigned jobs in hospitals in different cities, finally settling in *Hándān, Héběi* Province (see Figure 2.1). Ms *Tao* attended women having various kinds of difficult labour and soon became skilful in her job. Being a birth attendant was a route for her to become a midwife and then an obstetrician. She learned her art and science by actually doing midwifery, observing and assisting the senior staff in a variety of locations. Having served in a number of hospitals and received further training, the health system she served made full use of her remarkable attainments. She was promoted to be a midwife, an obstetrician and then a consultant obstetrician after a year or so of further training and an examination.

She was now able to perform five obstetric operations: forceps deliveries, caesarean section, cystoplasty (repair of the bladder), hysterectomy and hystero-oophorectomy. She talked about many techniques she had learned in her jobs, for example, altering the labouring woman's position to where the woman felt most comfortable and external and internal version to correct transverse lie.

In 1969 Ms *Tao* could no longer work in the hospitals because of a political purge. Instead, she had to work as a nursery nurse. Though she was a midwife herself, she gave birth to her first child unassisted, her second birth was attended by her husband and the last birth was by caesarean. She considered her birthing experience was much better than that of her mother and grandmother. Her mother gave birth to six babies, all the births being unassisted except for the first. Her grandmother had given birth unassisted to 14 children, with only three surviving and all the others dying at birth. That was in the late 19th and the early 20th centuries. This reminds us of an old Chinese saying 'A child is born anyway even if there is no assistance' (*jiēshēng, jiēshēng, bù jiē yě shēng*). The saying indicates Ms *Tao*'s belief in the natural process of childbirth, on one hand, and the professional relevance of midwifery, on the other, because without midwifery assistance, 11 of her grandmother's babies died at birth. Ms *Tao*'s personal story also supported her belief in the importance of midwifery, as she believes that midwifery has been an important part of social life in all major 'civilised' societies.

Rehabilitated and due to hospitals being short-staffed, she was recalled from being a nursery nurse to work as an obstetrician again. Opportunities also came for further study in a provincial hospital and, hence, promotion. She continued to work in *Hándān*, where she put her further learning into practice and even published several papers.

In 1997 Ms *Táo* ventured to The Congo twice to provide obstetrical services there, but she fractured her clavicle in a car accident. She received multiple honours and medals for her commitment in the services she provided for the Congolese people but received naught for her injuries. Ms *Táo* had to open her own clinic to earn money on returning home. Because of her failing health, she closed her clinic, but people still looked to her for services because of her reputation and people's trust.

Ms *Táo*'s achievements were surely due to her hard work, determination and commitment to her life goals and career as a maternity care provider. Her unsettled life witnessed the turbulent changes of 20th-century China. Here again, midwifery practice seemed just to be one step on the ladder leading to obstetric medicine, as there was no career development in midwifery alone.

However, the story of this self-taught humane and kindly obstetrician may naturally cause an interest and speculation in maternity care regulations in the country at that time.

A thoroughly modern midwife

In 2008 we interviewed Ms P., a highly influential figure in midwifery in an extremely prestigious province. Her career began auspiciously when she was sponsored to study nursing and awarded a BSc degree by a non-mainland Chinese university. Since then she has accumulated experience in obstetric and gynaecological care.

Ms P. attended Nursing School in 1979, when the school reopened after a 27-year break. In 1952 most industries and social services were being reinstated to where they had been in 1936 before the Sino-Japanese War (Geelan et al. 1974). Presumably, no or very little midwifery training existed during this period. According to Ms P., the political interruptions and upheavals affecting midwifery training after 1952 included the First Five Year Plan (1953–1957), the Great Leap Forward (1958–1962), and the Cultural Revolution (1966–1976). Midwifery education was a victim of these social and political upheavals. As mentioned in Chapter 3, Chinese midwifery was becoming modernised from 1928 when the European medical model was incorporated into Chinese practice. The modernisation of Chinese midwifery since 1928 might have improved birthing women's well-being; however, interruptions by wars and political upheavals disrupted its modernisation.

Due to her imagination and curiosity after observing a village birth, Ms P. developed a long-standing interest in midwifery and did well in her entrance examination. The acceptance of her application to the Nursing School stirred up a surge of interest in her village because it had never had a midwifery student before. Her success was seen as an achievement for the whole village. But the villagers' feelings were mixed, admiring the formal education she was to receive, yet loyal to the traditional professionals such as midwives, the *chăn-pó*. The formal state education seemed to have changed into one embodying the advance of science and technology to improve her social mobility. It was this transformation by a midwifery apprenticeship in the name of the nation state that motivated Ms P. to become a midwife.

Ms P. worked in labour ward for more than ten years and was promoted to Sister. While there her main interest was in learning obstetric interventions, such as using obstetric forceps, vacuum extraction and caesarean. She stressed many times in her interview that being able to learn and use these skills was the source of her motivation and inspiration for her work in the labour ward. She told us that she believed that her knowledge of obstetric techniques would enhance her professional confidence and status. For her, midwifery *per se* was not highly regarded.

Her focus on obstetric interventions led Ms P. to encourage similar attitudes in the midwifery staff. On the basis of this management style, she was appointed the Director of the province's Nursing Association in 2007. One year later a UK-trained midwife was persuaded to assist with the establishment of the mainland China's first midwifery association in the same province. On the basis of this midwifery association, Ms P. was able to consolidate her advancement, again with the same help, by achieving membership of the International Confederation of Midwives (ICM), another first in mainland China. This was not publicised, though, because colleagues in Shanghai warned her of possible political repercussions because of Taiwan's pre-existing ICM membership.

Clearly, Ms P.'s primary allegiances were not to midwifery or to the childbearing women who use midwifery services. This orientation became apparent in an income-generation exercise which promoted 'doula' services in her province. In this way, labour ward nurses known as 'midwives' undertook continuing education to expand doula services for wealthy, privileged clients at 'high-end' maternity services, serving to support the medicalisation of birth. The doula as a form of income generation was soon imitated throughout China.

A further step in her inexorable rise to power took the form of Ms P. requesting to host the Normal Labour and Birth Conference in 2012. Her involvement was more as a figurehead than making any active contribution. The catalogue of this midwife's relentless rise continued when she became the chairperson of the newly established 'Midwives Sub-branch' under the Chinese Maternal and Child Health Association in 2015.

To chronicle Ms P.'s meteoric career development is to demonstrate how midwifery may be used in modern China for purely personal rewards, without recognising the needs of or implications for midwives and childbearing women.

Midwifery scholars: debate and prospects

The issues identified in the interviews with 12 midwifery leaders and/or academics were the scholarship, leadership, debates and prospects in midwifery. Figure 10.3 shows an interview with two of these 12 midwifery leaders and academics before their first celebration of the International Midwives day organised by Ms *Chén Xiăohé* and firmly supported by Ms *Xióng Yŏngfāng on* 5 May 2009 in China. The summary of the authors' understanding of and reflection on the stories told by these people are presented in four sections below. The intention is to illuminate many unexplained incidents in Chinese midwifery history.

Scholarship

The consensus from our respondents is that for thousands of years, midwives or *chăn-pó* in China have provided care to birthing women and have formed an important part of Chinese civilisation. They are content that up until now,

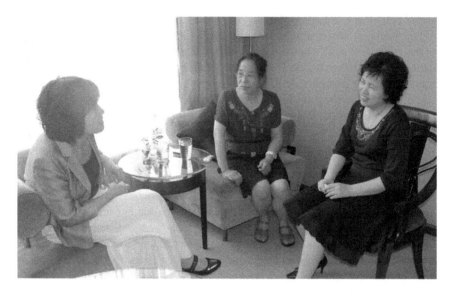

Figure 10.3 The interview in *Shēnzhèn* with two midwifery leaders Ms *Chén Xiǎohé* (left; *Shēnzhèn*) and Ms *Xióng Yǒngfāng* (right; *Wǔhàn*) before the first celebration of International Midwives Day organised and supported by them in the country in 2009

Source: Photograph by the authors' assistant.

midwifery practice has never constituted a serious subject of scholarly investigation. Indeed, midwifery is now still absent from the disciplines in the university enrolment in China. It is seemingly believed that to help a woman to give birth to a baby and to care for both of them before and after the birth may just involve some practical skills. These skills have disparagingly been compared to those required of a mechanic, who looks after an engine, as the 'mechanistic view point of giving birth' (Oakley 1980: 35; Wagner E.D. 1994), but are not dissimilar from a surgeon's skills. If surgeons' and physicians' discipline comprises medical knowledge, midwives must have theirs in the well-being of birthing women, the cultures, the societies and the individuals who give birth. All these and other aspects of caring and attending births would make up the subject matter that could place midwifery in higher education as an intellectual equal to other academic disciplines.

Leadership

A total of 12 respondents to our interviews were in national positions of authority at different levels. The leadership skills they presented in their stories were of three kinds: hierarchical, industrial and transformational (Byrom et al. 2011).

Hierarchical leadership values the culture of absolute top-down authority and control. Industrial leadership frames authoritarian leadership to influence the behaviour or action of other people within their positions and personality. Last, but not least, transformational leadership stands against autocratic and hierarchical styles, by stressing the development of positive self-esteem, and a focus on people to stimulate their feelings of elevation to become leaders themselves.

Autocratic leaders are indeed marvellous at understanding the intentions of their superiors. Their utterances, however, often show little power of thought, nor familiarity with philosophy and science other than fashionable current sayings and deeds. An example from their stories illustrates their leadership characteristics by having closed-circuit television and cardiotocograph monitoring systems in labour rooms to observe the work of staff and the progress of women in labour. This round-the-clock online surveillance depersonalises maternity care, violates the privacy of women and removes any trust between them and the staff. It obviously shows no depth to their thinking, but their supercilious authority, resting on contempt for women and staff.

The dominant type of leadership observed in our study is industrial leadership, which appears to influence the behaviour or action of other people within their positions and personality. Leadership of this style appears to be moving away from dictatorial authority or hierarchical models of direct command and control and moving towards those based on human relationships.

Finally, 'transformational' leaders include those working in the midwife-led normal birth unit in *Hángzhōu* (see Chapter 5; Cheung & Fleming 2011. Although they are the minority, they are working hard to try to overcome midwives' tendency to be directive. They are facilitating and supporting clinical staff to provide woman-centred care. Simultaneously, they empower those who are capable to become leaders to influence midwifery services at local and national levels. This leads to a question of their motive. No doubt, this group of leaders were not inspired by need or greed. Perhaps it was their desire to find their identity and to do things differently.

The capabilities and quality of Chinese midwifery leaders determine the direction and progression of Chinese midwifery in China. As it stands, it still needs time and further education for them to move away from a hierarchical to a flexible and relevant woman-centred care model.

Debates

Although a lack of midwifery leadership has been well acknowledged in China (Chang & Lu 2013), there is a growing body of knowledge in relation to what matters to mothers, midwives and obstetricians. This is resulting in a challenge to medical leadership in maternity care. The twelve midwifery leaders we interviewed stated that they are obliged to follow current medical models in the hope of getting medical help in return to develop their own capabilities and expand the body of midwifery leaders.

Midwifery as a significant academic discipline only emerged in major industrial countries in the late 20th century, while in some others midwifery practice was still not regulated and even outlawed. Following the move of midwifery into higher education, both undergraduate and postgraduate degree courses have been offered at universities since the 1990s. This development has provided new perspectives for Chinese academics to see midwifery as a profession, especially after the ICM Gap Analysis Workshop (GAW) in 2014 in *Shíjiāzhuāng*, China (see Chapter 5). Yet it looks at the moment, as if there is a long way to go before establishing midwifery as an academic discipline in Chinese universities. It is foreseeable, though, that through research and debate, the academic discipline of midwifery will eventually develop in China. It is also worth bearing in mind that multidisciplinary approaches are now increasingly apparent in academia worldwide. Such approaches have greatly expanded the scope of scholarly pursuit in higher education, a direction for midwifery to follow.

Indeed, why should there be any doubt? We have been studying Chinese midwifery as insiders and outsiders over the past two decades. We have witnessed the low and high of the development of Chinese midwifery. Maternity care in China has become hierarchical, with a ladder to climb from birth attendant to obstetrician under the shadow of medical science and technology (as discussed earlier in this chapter). Those who now hold positions in maternity care management or education had their days as birth attendants, nurses and/or midwives, working while learning. Now, as elites in the maternity care provision in China, they generally have to have positive attitudes towards midwifery education, advocating midwives as a power group and as a professional force in providing care to women throughout the birthing process.

However, we observed that prominent professionals in maternity care in China had a public version for our study and, for posterity, another private history. They are generally blessed with maternity care expertise through a medical channel, but they still see daily the abuse of caesarean section, the higher rate of which has caused concern among observers within and outside China (Cheung et al. 2005a, b; Renfrew et al. 2014).

Further questions for them to answer were, 'In what way midwives would become a power group and a professional force in maternity care?' and 'What is the essence of the concern about caesarean rates?' Their answer to both questions lay in the framework of what we call 'normal birth', but some of them sighed over the golden time when midwives could still attend births and prescribe/administer medicines. However, we were told that the pendulum may soon swing back to address the problematic status of midwifery and obstetrics' role in birth in China.

There were negative opinions among the top academics in this group of respondents, though. These opinions held that it was unlikely that midwives would ever make care decisions. They argued that medical science had provided the only framework to which midwives had recourse. Here it looked that for many, physiological science, which could be crucial to midwifery practice, had always been manipulated by obstetric medicine. It would then be very difficult to distinguish health from pathology, obstetric medicine's original *raison d'être*. So, it was argued, when decisions were made, being pathological or normal, the necessity of medical science was fundamental. It was argued that women always sought assurance from doctors, but not midwives and that women had more confidence in doctors than in midwives. It was thought so prevalent that people often would think that nurses and/or midwives were doctors, and they were very happy to be addressed as such because this was perceived by them as a positive sign of trust and respect from their clients. That had created the impression that doctors were in short supply in maternity, but midwives were not.

It is little wonder that midwives should be redundant from the verdicts these scholars introduced. There was clearly an obsession among them with 'risk' and 'uncertainty' in birthing, around which medical science centred, to such an extent that medical technology should be used irrespective of whether it is needed. The logical consequence was that midwives were only needed when high risk and uncertainty were absent. Thus, it appeared that the risk of a poor outcome would determine the course of action rather than choosing a course leading to the desired outcome. A logical extension of this would go as far as to stipulate that only doctors hold the licence to practise, even under normal circumstances.

So under the frame of 'risk' and 'uncertainty', midwifery training has become irrelevant and when facing the problem of maintaining midwifery education, the first question would be 'What could midwives do in a business as risky as having babies?' This is very different from the question, 'What could midwives do to improve what they have done for thousands of years for childbearing women?' As the decision was now being made in the name of the nation state, it was politically important, but it could turn into a political hot potato. Therefore, caution could be the best policy.

Under a medical regime, they, as high-profile nursing-midwifery professionals, could not agree that midwives held the key to reducing the caesarean rate since these were medical decisions. Additionally, other more complex social factors operate, such as women's choice, the birthing culture (where people chose auspicious dates for the birth), the media, people's belief in the technology and so on. If doctors are that decisive, then it is more likely the caesarean rate will rise rather than fall, for who can persuade those who have been trained to use the knife to lay it down? One may argue that it is a matter of encouraging or discouraging its use. But one can also ask whether the knife is needed at all. There was irony, though, when it was cited that it was often labour delivery room nurses/midwives who suggested caesareans; their reason being that they could no longer cope with the workload.

Prospects

Now we have other more complex factors and they are so diverse that the way ahead appears long and arduous. Of all these variables, there is one thing that is constant, that is that care should be provided. Women may not make choices, people do not believe in lucky dates any more, and the media have changed the fashion, and so on, but care is still needed. Now the carers are the doctors and the nurses. If doctors and nurses are unable to solve the problem, then it must be the midwives who have long held the key to natural, healthy, satisfying births. For the midwives to do so competently, a framework is needed in contradistinction to the obstetric model. We see this is a framework of 'normal birth'. To substantiate this framework is exactly the core of midwifery.

The respondents all agreed that a framework of 'normal birth' opens up immense possibilities for midwifery. This proposal immediately suggests a woman-centred approach, implying individual care, because 'normality' is essential to the woman who is rooted in her own natural, social and cultural environment. If this is the case, then midwifery will be constantly searching to understand different forms of birth. The academic repertoire of midwifery can then be filled with these cases, an approach not dissimilar to that of modern medical practice, but in opposition to the concept of pathology. We can also envisage a theoretical midwifery, incorporating multidisciplinary themes, methods and approaches in alliance with other disciplines in health and in social science. These prospects can now be brought forward in discussion with midwifery professionals in China and elsewhere who have maintained that the quality of student training lay in their ability to handle the literature. The fruit of science, the literature is an unquestionably authoritative access to the profession. Any break with this tradition was considered out of place. It is true that the literature has summarised predecessors' professional experiences and provided a learning resource. But how this fruit of science is bitten will be more important than just biting it.

To transform midwifery education, the scope and the methods of teaching and learning have to be widened, involving both research and clinical experience. Unfortunately, midwifery texts have been so immersed in medical science that midwifery students have become hardened by a framework, parts of which were laid down half a century ago. A regulatory framework may be the scientific product as they are told, but it is also the product of our own experience across time and space. From this perspective, such a framework can only be enriched through continuous research and experience, so that midwifery students will not want to quibble over the timing of stages of labour, the measurements of cervical dilation, and so on. In some recent developments, some of the respondents argued that teaching in a discipline like midwifery, resorting to the scientific evidence-based research are insufficient. The students' and teachers' intuition and experience will play equally important roles in education (Walsh 2007a, b). That would represent a step forward.

Nursing-midwifery professionals in China, especially those in the key universities among our respondents, may have been enmeshed within the medical scientific agenda for too long; resulting in the feeling that it was somebody 'up there', not us, who could create the regulatory framework. The best they could do was to adhere to these regulations. That could be objective enough, but one cannot help asking whether there is some truth in the adage that 'rules and regulations are there to break'. Of course, here it is not in the sense of breaking away; it is in the sense of breaking forward.

Discussion: social and economic status

Studying the interactions of a childbirth carer and interpreting her ideas brings us close to her, her social psychology and her profession.

What are we to make of these stories?

Seven kinds of carers were included among our respondents, despite the technological modernisation and health authorities' constant efforts to eradicate midwifery practice. They are

1   traditional midwives,
2   modern birth attendants,
3   midwives,
4   nurse-midwives,
5   nurse-midwife teachers,
6   self-taught midwife-obstetricians and
7   midwife-academics.

Some of them practised on an occasional basis and attended only a small number of births. Others, practising more regularly gained respect and cooperation from the local health workers. These are a contentious form of evidence. They are controversial because the respondents are still alive, and the issue of their identity as midwives is still being debated in China, not to mention the other issues of professionalisation, marginalisation and modernisation of midwifery.

The traditional midwife respondents in our study were wives or widows of doctors, artisans or peasants, who were wealthy enough to own their own houses (as discussed earlier in this chapter). When they started to practise midwifery, they had already given birth. On one hand, they found themselves respectable, in a position of having a high level of esteem and social mobility because of their social and economic positions. On the other hand, they tended to stay in the rural and urban slum areas. They developed a commitment to their fellow country-women. These women used their services and at the same time these traditional midwives also learned from the women their stories of happiness, sorrow and death. These kindled their ambition and gave them an opportunity to serve people, as well as making their living.

The modern midwives, nurse midwives, nurse-midwife teachers and midwife teachers were college graduates and became public salaried employees. They were often women of considerable social status and central figures in terms of childbirth in the local community. Most of them worked in big hospitals or teaching institutions, but as midwifery was still in a dubious position in Chinese maternity care, intra-professional communication and exchange were almost non-existent. Since the beginning of this century, however, some national and regional midwifery or nursing training or research conferences have been convened. These gatherings of midwives, or obstetric nurses, have revealed a lack of new research and little exchange of new thinking that could be generated from the clinical experience of the midwives. To a large extent, these gatherings were training classes in which new copies of older midwifery textbooks, from as far back as the 1950s or 1960s, were still being used unquestioningly and taken as standard.

There was nevertheless a general aspiration for new information, particularly at the international gatherings. This is in sharp contrast to the lack of active communication based on the research by midwives themselves. This lack of communication led to a tendency among the midwives to form professional groups, which could be observed in these conferences. There were differences in their approaches to the medical model of childbirth, with midwives based in bigger cities adhering more to the medical hierarchy and those in smaller ones showing resistance to such a model. While it was not surprising in such a big country as China that there should be differences, geographical, social or even economic, within the same profession, it posed questions for the future formation of this important public sector in China. A researching, exchanging and openly debating culture had yet to be created to replace other less relevant forms of professional grouping.

Evidence regarding midwives' social status demonstrates that, though midwifery itself is marginalised, midwives were not marginalised in their communities. This is particularly true of traditional midwives, who provide home births and care when the families do not care if the birth can be registered or not, while modern midwives provide care in the public domain.

Chinese midwives' stories are about their communities, education, choices, successes, failures and constraints on their actions. Most of them are employed in developed areas where the practice of birth attendants is widely condemned officially; maternity care has come to be dominated by doctors with nearly all births taking place in hospitals. The others are in less- or under-developed areas, where their community sets frameworks within which they live, work and make decisions. This has not only reflected the principal values and unequal social arrangements but also informed us of the devalued or marginal status of midwifery.

Hearing the stories of midwives who experienced the common and uncommon events of Chinese midwifery enlivens the historical narrative. We listened to not only what we were told but, more important, to the ideas that the stories could carry as well. We tried to look beyond the event and ideas to see how the midwives stood in the context and in relation to others in the profession.

The experiences of a midwifery practitioner have been brought to light for the first time in this study, revealing the ideas and social exchanges that are all real between the practitioners and their clients, and in things themselves. They are, as a social phenomenon, the product of time and place. The respondents of this study appear now to be beginning to realise the limits and the impact of modern obstetric technology on their quality of life. More and more of them are becoming aware of something needing to be done, though, they are not so sure of what, when, where, how or by whom.

Although people work under the same political system, they demonstrate drastic differences. For example, the modern midwife Ms P. (as discussed earlier in this Chapter) looked up to obstetric technology. She was anxious to know the details of anything new in the sense of modern technological development and proud of being able to handle them. She is more inclined to accept and rely on a medical risk orientation. As to the basic midwifery nurturing skills, she overlooked them except for 'doula' services which are considered profitable for her and her institution. The role of a midwife as defined by the WHO (1999a, b) to assist physiological birth was virtually obscured in her story as childbirth became more hospital-based, medicalised and economically oriented. The midwives of her world increasingly adopted the new obstetric technical skills and the role of technical obstetric nurses or obstetricians. This made sense in China where technology was perceived as a symbol of modernisation, and their understanding was filtered through the lens of this concept. This calls for a more complicated theory and education model to address the complexity of the human beings and their behaviour. Ms P.'s story provides an insight into the life of a midwife showing her imagination, professional development, growth and success, which are inseparable from her personality and that personality, in itself, was complete, coherent and self-calculating. However, her understanding, beliefs and deeds are shaped by the existing medical care system. That is why she has been promoted to a responsible position, mouthpiece for the media and professor in a key university.

The traditional midwives and birth attendants interviewed in the study worked quietly in their communities. They were mature married or widowed women who started to practise when they had families. All of them had some kind of connection with medical clinics or health workers. They practised midwifery by learning through doing. Though their practice of midwifery was not necessarily imperative for the family income, it was a useful addition. Despite the fact that they received no recognition from the authorities, their services in the community appeared to be vital to the health and welfare of women and babies. They very often enjoyed popularity and respect in their communities.

The modern nurse-midwives in our study were familiar with obstetric technologies. They were ordinary working women, wage earners with a sense of pride in their profession. Their roles were much wider than the art of midwifery. They often overlooked the midwifery skills and accepted modern interventions and technologies. The respected midwifery academics in their circles expressed strongly in their interviews that they were happy to accept what they were told and lacked interest in the challenge which came from their students and the development of Chinese midwifery. These changes in their attitude were subtle, slower and more complex than we realised.

We believe that this study of the present lives of Chinese midwives is able to improve our understanding of the status and quality of historical knowledge. We hope to provide a true account of Chinese midwives and midwifery. What do we mean by a true account? One aspect of this answer must be the highest possible levels of accuracy and precision, which is the purpose of this book and may suggest some alternative or prospect for the future. The further analyses and studies are concluded in the next chapters.

11　Does China need midwifery?

Our examination of the development of Chinese midwifery in this book, the review of the documents of the Chinese Ministry of Health and National Health and Family Planning Commission (NHFPC) (see Further Reading and Notes – Midwifery policies in China) and the findings of the International Confederation of Midwives (ICM) gap analysis workshop (GAW) (see Further Reading and Notes – The International Confederation of Midwives Gap Analysis Workshop in China) help us to understand and write about the present situation. The comparison between the past and present facilitates our understanding of how and why Chinese midwifery and its practitioners have become social, economic and professional casualties. This may lead to questions about what is the present and when does the past end and the present begin. Our basic understanding is that the concepts of present and past are constructed by us, as human beings. What happened prior to the issue under discussion is the past. Knowing its past then helps us understand the present position now and to predict and shape its future. To break out of this past will require not only historical knowledge and awareness but also, more important, a recognition of its development in the wider context to make sense of the here and now.

The international development of midwifery takes place in the context of health systems in high-income countries. Ideally, commitment to universal access to some form of midwifery for all women and families would promote the well-being of their citizens and realise greater social equality for its population (UNFPA 2011, 2014; Renfrew et al. 2014). The macro world view of midwifery development may aid people to question whether China needs midwifery to care for its population.

It is easy to forget that what happens in Chinese maternity care is a product of state policies, which influence everything from state policy decisions, through interactions between care providers and clients to clinical outcomes. The case of China allows us an opportunity to examine the social organisation of maternity care and state involvement in maternity health policy.

Maternity care in hospitals and village clinics

The accounts in this section are taken from our interviews during our fieldwork in the past decade.

In hospitals

In 2012, we visited a pre-labour area in a key public hospital in central northern China. The room was about 30 square metres, and there were more than a dozen pregnant women sitting along one wall with intravenous oxytocin to expedite labour; three women were lying on beds along the opposite wall with fetal monitors attached.

'We have to do this routinely because we are really running short of hands', the ward sister explained; 'we have more than 10,000 deliveries annually but only 60 staff'. Such an arrangement of a pre-labour area may not be typical throughout China. As China's economy continues to grow, families have been allowed a second child since 2015; there is no doubt that bigger maternity wards are now being built to cope with the extra demand anticipated.

In fact, hundreds and thousands of private luxurious maternity hospitals are mushrooming as products of the government's strategy to provide 'high-end' maternity care to target the rich, the privileged and those who have medical insurance. The 'high-end' private hospitals we visited include the following:

1   Shanghai Redleaf International Women and Children's Hospital (上海红枫国际妇儿医院) built by Chinese Canadians in 2013
2   United Family Hospitals (和睦家医院), a registered US charity operating in China since 2001 under the auspices of the United Foundation for China's Health
3   Baijia Maternity Care Holdings (百佳妇婴健康产业控股集团, BMCH 2014) established in 2011 aiming to create a chain of 100 hospitals in the metropolises around the country

These private hospitals have been regarded as the leaders in the state policy of China Medical Reform. They are the pace-setters for Chinese women and infants medical care to transform the '10-month pregnancy' into 12 months, and to transform maternity services to hotel services and/or medical tourism.

One of the 'low-end' hospitals we visited in 2013 in *Ānhuī* Province was a modern maternity hospital with more than 2,000 births annually. As there was only one labour bed it was difficult for us to comprehend how the hospital coped with such a workload. That was until we were told that their annual caesarean rate was well over 60%. The caesarean rates of the nine state-owned hospitals we visited in *Ānhuī*, *Sìchuān* and *Shǎnxī* Provinces in the same year were well over 40% at level 1 (district) hospitals and 70% to 80% at level 2 and 3 hospitals in big cities.

The 'low-end' maternity service providers are mainly those public hospitals owned by the state. It appears strange for the central health policy-makers to allow most of the health resources to be directed to serve the rich and privileged few and less for the public. This practice appears to go against the philosophy upheld by the socialist or communist government to serve members of the public. However, this well-known paradox has caught our concern as this logic appears to have driven the primary health care provided by these public hospitals into ruin: in that it is downgraded to be low-end service providers in fierce competition with the private hospitals.

Midwifery care has also been segmented and transformed into different commodities, such as 'doula' services during labour/birth, *'yuèsǎo* postnatally, and *'xiǎo-ā-huá'* (Guide – Chinese glossary) for breast feeding support; none of the staff, however, had been appropriately trained and assessed for their jobs. All services being offered were dependent on the women's ability to pay, but not necessarily related to their needs. The women's health insurance and inpatient delivery payments did not cover these services. In this way the maternity service providers were transformed into the munificent benefactors of privatisation of their services. Although a poster listing the rights of women (WHO 2007) was displayed in some hospitals, no one seemed to bother to understand or refer to women's rights.

In village clinics

Village clinics were discouraged from providing maternity services by the government; this was because they were not allowed to issue birth certificates if a birth took place there. These clinics only accepted those women without a birth permission or not intending to register the birth. During our visit to a village clinic near *Xīān* (see Figure 2.1, Map of China), a mother-in-law came to request the traditional midwife to attend her daughter-in-law's birth, but she was advised to take her daughter-in-law to a level 2 or 3 hospital if the birth of that child needed to be registered.

Although all women interviewed in another study (Cheung & Pan 2012) had planned to give birth vaginally, more than half of them could not. What happened to them? Why did so many of them need a caesarean? What are the consequences for women and their babies as a result? The answers to these questions are under investigation in another ongoing study.

Case study: the disrespect of midwifery in China

The first alongside midwife-led normal birth unit (MNBU) was developed through an international collaborative action research project in 2008 (see Chapter 5), in response to the increasing number of unnecessary caesareans and the diminishing role of midwives. The midwife-led care (MLC) was tailored to the needs and the circumstances of women during childbirth. There was immediately great demand from women and families. The chief investigator was approached after the success of the initiative by the heads and managers of 14 hospitals, who requested seminars and visits to help them develop MNBUs in their hospitals throughout the country. In response to these requests, a comparative randomised controlled trial (RCT) was designed and incorporated into the four-year COST Action IS0907 project (see Chapter 5). It was 'the Midwife-led Care Study – the development and exploration of the effectiveness of midwife-led services in 10 hospitals in China'.

The aim was to improve maternal and perinatal well-being for healthy women and babies at term by reducing caesarean rates from 40% to 30% through the implementation of MNBUs.

The objectives were

1   to establish midwife-led units in 10 Chinese hospitals;
2   to set up a randomised controlled trial to assess the impact of MNBUs;
3   to develop these sites as research centres for future programmes of study throughout the country.

The long-term goal was to maximise well-being for childbearing women and their children through the elimination of inappropriate intrapartum interventions.

The project was eventually approved and funded by *Hángzhōu* Human Resources and Social Security Bureau, *Zhèjiāng* Province, China (the approval document number is [2013] No. 377). The midwives and medical staff from these hospitals were recruited, trained and prepared for the project for over a year.

Just as it was about to start, the project was suddenly brought to a halt. An unexpected changeover of all the senior university staff, where the first author worked, followed a corruption investigation and the arrest of the vice president. The new leaders pursued different agendas and visions. The nursing school was merged with the medical school. The funds earmarked for this RCT study and the ICM Gap Analysis Workshop (see Chapter 5) were redirected. Again, midwifery was being perceived as expendable. Both crucial midwifery projects were thus terminated by ignorant newcomers. Although the ICM GAW was eventually held successfully, albeit with great difficulty and effort in *Shíjiāzhuāng* city, *Héběi* Province, the RCT was abandoned as too great an undertaking for the community of Chinese midwives to carry out unaided.

Midwives in Ministry of Health policies

A total of 63 out of 1189 CMoH documents since 1949 (see Further Reading and Notes – Midwifery policies in China) related to maternity care and midwifery have been located during our research. They were retrieved and reviewed with reference to historical development, governance and the barriers to midwifery services. There were no specific regulations for midwifery or midwives. Only seven CMoH documents mentioned 'midwife', without any clear indication of its meaning: four before 1987, and three after 2008. Midwives in these documents were identified as either nurses or birth attendants and were treated as if they were expendable. Midwifery has thus been 'discouraged' nationally and total hospitalisation of childbirth promoted (People's Daily 2001, 2002; CMoH et al. 2003; Cheung 2009; Feng et al. 2011). Compliance with this national policy is closely scrutinised so that if goals for hospital births were not achieved, staff salaries would be cut (Harris et al. 2009b) and bonuses would be withheld. Clinical staff report experiencing frustration due to inadequate resources provided by central health authorities, staff incompetence and policy-makers' indifference.

All of this happened against the background of the prevalent birth control policies. As births became less important to society, so midwifery practice became more of a thing of the past. A 1986 document stipulated that a midwife's job was confined to the labour room and staff working in antenatal and postnatal areas were nurses. This document was eventually abolished together with the other six in 2011, without new relevant policies being put in place (CMoH 2011a). However, the management of midwives and maternity care have been subsumed under the central government's Department of Nursing and Medicine.

These documents led us to view the concept of 'midwifery', from the policies of the CMoH and the NHFPC (see Further Reading and Notes – Midwifery policies in China) as the 'aid to delivery', such as assistance with forceps, ventouse or episiotomy. This was considered, by these documents, to concur with the global 'Safe Motherhood Initiative' (World Bank et al. 1987), which was interpreted in China as an effort to enhance national and local facility-based maternity care. As a result, the statistics showed that unnecessary interventions were soaring and a shift was needed from an interventive approach to a more holistic system of care. In the eyes of policy-makers, 'midwifery' implies customary, normal, natural or physiological birth, and therefore, it conveys a sense of simple and 'untechnical' interventions. It was discouraged and, paradoxically, obstetric technologies are now being promoted in order to assume total control (CMoH 2009).

Imbalance of midwives and obstetricians

Although China had its first state-owned midwifery school in 1928 and now has an annual birth rate of about 17 million, midwifery has been stopped from developing in the past 40 years (Cheung 2009). In 1975, there were about 87,700 obstetricians in China. By 2011, the number had reached 435,100 (CMoH 2012), a five-fold increase, while the population had merely doubled. It was also during these four decades that China implemented the world's most ruthless one-child birth control policy, which alone reduced the workload, perceived as burdensome, on maternity services. There is no doubt that these developments and changes have meant greater improvement in maternal and infant health to a large extent. Statistically, China claimed to have achieved its Millennium Development Goal in reducing maternal mortality by 2015. This is despite a serious shortage of carers, even though more doctors are trained and fewer babies are now born and the prevalence of caesareans as shown earlier in this chapter.

'Midwives' in China nowadays are registered nurses and doctors working in labour rooms with two to four years of basic college or undergraduate nursing education and three months labour ward clinical experience (Pang 2010). Clinically, when increased caesarean use was condemned, midwives' jobs were extended to embrace induction and augmentation of labour and epidurals; also included was advice about IVF (in vitro fertilisation) to families hoping to give birth to twins to overcome the one-child policy. Some midwives, together with nurses, 'moonlight' as doula midwives to supplement their income.

There were 44,000 midwives and 227,000 birth attendants in China in 2000, according to the statistics of *Húzhōu* Women net (2008) and CMoH (2001). The number of midwives was reduced to 39,000 by 2010 (Pang 2010). The category of 'midwives' has disappeared from health care statistics since 2001 (CMoH 2001). Though some effort has been made since 2006, there has not been any undergraduate degree courses for midwifery yet, despite a co-operative alliance between Peking University and New Zealand's Waikato Institute of Technology (Wintec 2006) and some initiatives funded by the United Nations Children's Fund (UNICEF; see Chapter 6). There is no bachelor's degree in midwifery offered at any university. This clearly illustrates the attitude and the marginal position midwifery and midwives are in the maternity services and in education. The basic rights of women to access midwifery care are thus denied and replaced by medical care, which can be observed from the disproportionate numbers in the maternity health workforce (Figure 11.1).

The distribution of midwives in the maternity workforce was uneven. Most midwives were concentrated in labour wards in level 3 and 2 hospitals. Village- and community-level hospitals had no midwives. The six major barriers to the development of midwifery were identified in the ICM GAW and the discussions of its participants (see Chapter 5; Further Reading and Notes – The International Confederation of Midwives Gap Analysis Workshop in China – Gaps identified):

1   Absence of national regulations and standards
2   Absence of a national higher education system
3   Absence of a national midwives association
4   Absence of a career development ladder
5   Misconception of midwifery as a symbol of backwardness
6   A lack of understanding of 'normal birth' at the levels of women, health workers and maternity policy-makers

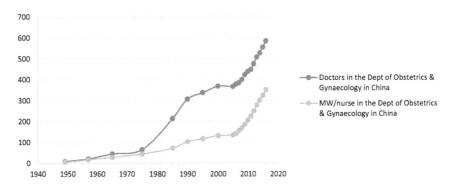

Figure 11.1 The numbers of obstetricians and midwives/nurses in maternity care in China
Sources: CMoH (1997–2012); Pang (2010); NBoSoC 2017.
Note: MW = midwife.

Midwives and midwifery in China have been linked to high mortality in resource-limited settings (People's Daily 2001). This was, in fact, not the fault of midwives; it was due to inadequate support for midwives in education and clinical practice for high-quality services because of the absence of a national policy, a national education system and a national professional body.

Chinese maternal, perinatal and neonatal mortality

The 'facility-based strategy' in China has been well intentioned, aiming for a reduction in maternal and perinatal mortality and morbidity. In interpreting the outcomes of this strategy, it is necessary to bear in mind the problem of counting the number of maternal deaths (Mander 2010). Keeping accurate statistics may not be a priority in under-resourced health care settings, and in some rural and remote areas, the childbearing woman who dies may not have been attended by a person sufficiently knowledgeable to report her death. This means that maternal mortality figures may depend, for example, on population-based estimates (Baraté & Temmerman 2009). Despite this caution, it is necessary for us to employ here the data which are available and a comparison of maternal mortality figures with previous decades reveals the limited success of this strategy, as Figure 11.2 shows.

While the published statistics show that China was able to reduce its maternal mortality from 15,000 per 100,000 live births in 1949 to 19.9 in 2016 (Figure 11.3), other figures reveal hidden problems.

The annual decline in the maternal mortality rate (MMR) in the 30-year period before 1980 was more significant (between 20% and 40%), when medicine was less well developed, than the equivalent period after 1980 (between 10% and

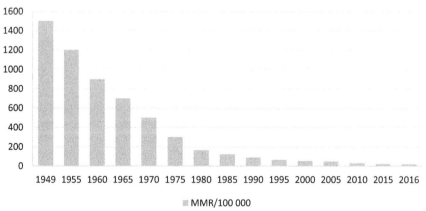

China's MMR from 1949-2016

Figure 11.2 Maternal mortality rate (MMR) in China, 1949–2016 (1:100,000)

Sources: Gapminder (2010); CMoH (2012); NHFPC (2016, 2017); NBoSoC (2017).

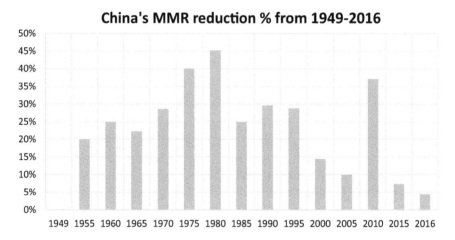

Figure 11.3 China's maternal mortality reduction (%), 1949–2016

Sources: Gapminder (2010); CMoH (2012); NHFPC (2016).

37%). The greatest decrease in the MMR was between 1970 and 1980 when China was in turmoil during the Cultural Revolution (see Chapter 8). This was when city doctors were sent to rural areas as a form of political punishment, and unregulated traditional midwives were actively involved in maternity care (see Chapter 10). As a result, rural maternal health was improved, while using only 20% of national health care resources. Ironically 80% of maternity care resources were concentrated in cities caring for only 20% of the nation's population in the 1970s and the 1980s. Now, though, due to internal migration, around 60% of the population dwell in rural areas (CMoH et al. 2006b; Shen 2008; Cheung & Pan 2012).

Although such a decline in MMR was impressive from the perspective of hospitalisation of childbirth there, China was surprisingly lagging behind countries of lower economic development such as Sri Lanka and Vietnam (Lumbiganon et al. 2010).

The reduction of the perinatal mortality rate (PMR), neonatal mortality rate (NMR), infant mortality rate (IMR) and MMR from the 1990s, though, may present difficult concepts for some Chinese researchers (see Figure 11.4). These have led to some undesirable confusions and misunderstandings in their findings and papers. However, the issue of IMR appears to be better understood. In *Huáng*'s study (2016), a total of 68% of infant mortality was found to be failing to be declared in the sixth every-ten-year national population census in 2010. The official figures (CMoH 2010; NHFPC 2013, 2016) are much lower than the 2010 census. Disregarding the missing figures in the census (*Huáng* 2016), the falls in these rates, reflecting improvements in maternal and child health, were limited. Significantly, they lagged behind many Asian countries at a similar or

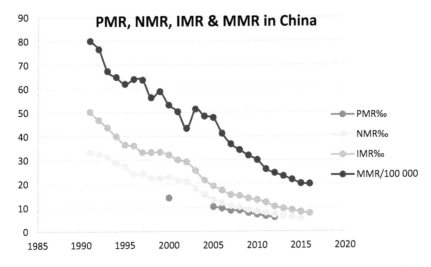

Figure 11.4 Perinatal, neonatal, infant and maternal mortality rates in China, 1991–2015

Sources: CMoH (2010); NHFPC (2013, 2016).

Notes: PMR: perinatal mortality rate

NMR: neonatal mortality rate

IMR: infant mortality rate

MMR: maternal mortality rate

even lower level of economic development than China (Pang 2010; Souza et al. 2010; Lumbiganon 2010).

These figures, especially the MMR, have not really kept pace with the economic growth and the increase in hospital births. Thus, we can argue that the current 'facility-based' birth care does not necessarily hold the key to improve maternal and infant health. Rather, accessibility and availability of services are crucial.

The facility-based strategy has largely been compromised by social inequality in economic development. It has been revealed that in this era of economic development, more and more skilled birth attendants are giving up attending births but are performing caesareans. They are increasingly spending their time handling and maintaining equipment and recording data in charts. The system is making normal birth difficult to achieve. Women and families tend to be regarded as potential adversaries in a lawsuit, and health workers are enslaved by machinery that was once used to save lives.

Discussion: implications for practice

In the main, our study is based on the review of the practices and issues of Chinese midwifery, the CMoH documents, and the findings of the surveys and discussions of the ICM GAW. It takes the development of midwifery and the controversial policy options in China into a debate with the goal of reinstating midwives in midwifery care to enhance midwifery and improve the health of women, babies and families there.

China has not had better maternal outcomes, in the past 30 years despite its fast economic development and increasing medical facilities. The evidence collected shows that economic growth alone will not deliver good health outcomes. The challenges of the market economy in maternity care has driven the maternity services to put more emphasis on users' fees, and income generation; as a result, more and more unnecessary treatments and operative deliveries are being carried out instead of providing high-quality midwifery care. The epidemic of caesareans, medical interventions, and inconsistent midwifery education, regulatory and management systems have resulted in poor-quality maternity care and near absence of normal birth. The key to breaking this vicious circle is to re-establish midwifery as a major component of the workforce; thus, normal labour and birth will revert to being a physiological family-building process, and health and family care will be reintegrated.

The barriers identified were the absence of regulations pertaining to midwives at the macro level, the invisibility of midwifery and its services at the meso level and the confinement of midwives in the labour wards at the micro level. These analyses show that Chinese midwifery needs to become accepted in higher education. Additionally, midwives need to have their own national association in order to have a strong voice in health policy to ensure women can access them and their high-quality services.

The evidence and debate suggest the following conclusions:

1   Midwives were the main carers during childbearing and childbirth in Chinese history. They were respected before the *Sòng* dynasty but gradually lost favour and disappeared in the late 20th century.
2   The evidence from the ICM GAW (see Further Reading and Notes – The International Confederation of Midwives Gap Analysis Workshop in China) shows the demise of midwives and midwifery is the direct result of the absence of specific regulations, higher education and a national association for midwives since 1949 in mainland China.
3   The policy of using obstetricians and nurses to replace midwives on the grounds of safety is not supported by the available evidence.
4   There is no evidence that morbidity and mortality are higher among mothers and babies cared by midwives.
5   A majority of women who had experienced midwife-led maternity services preferred to have midwives' services.
6   There is no evidence to support the claim that midwifery is backward.
7   No satisfactory explanation has been found to justify the demise of Chinese midwifery and the disappearance of midwives.

The development of midwifery in China is facing a policy challenge and reform of the maternity care system is much needed; this requires a national restructuring of the system. Such a challenge to Chinese capitalism would be made even more difficult by the current lack of general understanding of the role of midwifery, midwives and normal childbirth. Midwifery is a critical component of the maternity services that can resolve gaps in accessibility, acceptability, quality and efficiency of maternity services. Midwifery could be permanently responsible for safeguarding the physical and mental health and the well-being of mothers, newborns and their families in all societies. China, like countries throughout the world, needs midwifery and midwives.

There may be unavoidable tensions between eagerness for improvement, innovation of midwifery and the limits of evidence and resources. Such tensions threaten the ideal of woman-centred care within the pragmatic boundaries of maternal health systems and medical policies. To overcome these challenges national policy-makers will need to exercise all of their diplomatic functions in a spirit of reflection and humanity to protect the interests of the people. Success will demand courage and flexibility to challenge the diehards that would prevent the changes needed to bring about equity.

12 Epilogue

What do women want?

In our examination of midwifery in China, we have somehow failed to address how childbirth care has been provided for an individual there. The immediate question which arises is, 'What does a Chinese woman want?' Our historical and current studies suggest that a healthy, normal and uneventful birth as a family event is the desire of every woman. The choice an individual woman makes could be different. It is often made in accordance with her preference and/or that of her significant others, such as husband, in-laws and close friends. Her desires are thus shaped by her community, media and the existing maternity care system. Nothing we have found in the literature, so far, has fully addressed the complexity of the relationship between each woman's desire and maternity care, not to mention the task of meeting her needs and desires. However, it is possible that these can be addressed by an experienced competent midwife at a personal and practical level. The midwife, however, must respect and support the woman in her choices and decision, as well as recognise the natural rhythms of life before any intervention with the intention of improving it.

The experience of childbearing, during birth and in the early days and months afterwards, are perceived as crucially important for the well-being of the mother and her relationship with her child, her family and the wider society. These needs are what midwives have known throughout history, but in recent years have been unable to practise due to the imposition of medical efficiency and the demise of Chinese midwifery. Midwives nowadays have to negotiate constantly between the care system and their desires to help women to achieve their real choice. Further study is urgently needed for health workers to identify the who, what, where and why of a woman's wishes regarding her childbirth, bearing in mind the woman's need to enhance her sense of self and of self-worth within the family.

Though very challenging, the present book illustrates the influences and constraints that the wider society puts on Chinese midwifery, women and childbirth. We have addressed how state policy, educational institutions, professions and medical systems together with modern technology have shaped Chinese midwifery, maternity care and the desires of women. We have shown how women and midwives have become prisoners of the technology which has been created and which they feel compelled to use, one result of which has been women becoming victims of unnecessary and potentially iatrogenic obstetric interventions. Thus, childbirth has become a challenge both to the individual woman and to midwifery.

Development of Chinese midwifery

This book has taken up the issues of origin, characteristics and development of Chinese midwifery. The purpose has been, as we stated in Chapter 1, to find a way in which Chinese midwifery might be able to come to the fore to provide the care which women need and deserve in the future. The observations recounted here have helped us to see statements in context, and actions as they happen. In the process of this exploration and analysis, we have recovered the meanings, changing ideas and applications of Chinese midwifery in the following three major aspects.

First, the highs and lows of Chinese midwifery and the diverse experiences of Chinese midwives, though not conclusive, were introduced chronologically. Although Chinese Midwives Rules were established in 1928, the development of Chinese midwifery did not go very far in what people could expect. Childbirth was moved from the domestic sphere to the institutional domain with the missionaries' injection of Western medicine. The change in the place of birth from home to hospital has signalled a move of Chinese midwifery from physiological to medicalised childbirth, a development occurring in many western countries in the 1950s and 1960s with diminishing roles of midwives as a by-product of industrialisation due to a patriarchal culture. The imported obstetric model (Chapter 7) has questioned neither the definition of midwifery nor what counts as normal birth. As a result, midwifery has occupied a lower priority within the structure of health provision than obstetrics in China.

Second, the change of birth attendants from midwives to doulas, obstetric nurses and obstetricians was inevitably associated with changes in ideas and the development of technology. The shift in carers in childbearing and childbirth illuminates our perception of the arbitrariness of midwifery practice and helps us to see the inadequacy of Chinese midwives' roles and the limitations of obstetric care. The change of carers has contradictory and double-edged effects. The basic provision of essential information and the right to give birth without intervention were unavailable to women, especially for the poor. Obstetric care has become highly sought-after despite the high cost and the dangers associated with excessive and unnecessary interventions.

The decline of Chinese midwifery also highlights the inadequacy of central health policy and state legislation to protect the public interests. The policies have been questioned in the light of the evidence collected and the debate about the interpretation of midwifery and midwives in terms of professionalisation, modernisation and marginalisation. Our analysis shows that governments' appropriate policies are important in the workings of midwifery and of maternal and child health services. Leaving maternity services to the working of the free market means more interventions, more costs, and little chance to offer a better solution.

Third, the feelings, ideas, knowledges and lives of Chinese midwives have been presented as a social construct. Their lives and experiences are a reflection of their world which is largely nurtured and determined by society. However, the authors are also aware that no organisational framework alone can resolve all problems, and it is crucial to ensure a harmonious fit between the cultural context and the individual midwife.

The study of the lives and experiences of Chinese midwives in written materials has provided windows onto the past and led to a deeper understanding of the value of current Chinese midwives and the development of their profession. This has also highlighted the inequality between female-dominated midwifery and male-dominated obstetrics.

Currently ethical medical practice in China is problematic because of the present policy of a free-market economy. Midwifery is considered to be expendable, as technology or surgery are more profitable. The hospitals, obstetricians and nurses receive a financial incentive for each surgical operation performed. Women have been reduced, as Ann Oakley has argued, to the status of reproductive objects (Oakley 1976, 1987). We believe that our historical study can enable people to re-evaluate the pros and cons of midwifery in relation to obstetrics. The way to move forward is to serve the needs of women, babies and families, by respecting the decisions parents make about the birth of their children. True authority lies deep within the clients because they know what is best for them and what they can live with in their future.

The lives and work of Chinese midwives are both the product and they are the conscious or unconscious orators of the society to which they belong. Their past needs us to interpret and to make sense of it; without such an engagement of interpretation and reflection, the facts of what they did and experienced are unintelligible and dead. Our study recognises a new vision of and for Chinese midwifery, which is not only determined by history but also makes history. It shows how the arguments have advanced through these three aspects of this book.

Four emerging themes

Four themes have been emerging through this book. The first one is the role of women, in support of which the education and competence of midwives has been crucial in every period, especially in the informal care of childbirth. The evolution of their status and education is one of the major factors in the improvement of maternity care, as well as facilitating women's choice to have a normal and emotionally satisfying birth. Unfortunately, higher education for midwives is still in its formative stages, though the government has stated its intention to support it.

The second theme is the professionalisation of Chinese midwifery which is associated with the extension of the formal health care sector. Medicalisation and social control have been prominent, and Chinese midwifery has been fighting a losing battle relative to obstetrics; this is because of its low status as a second-class occupation since the *Sòng* dynasty (see Timeline) because of gender, propositional knowledge and technological choices. These attitudes persist, resulting in Chinese midwifery being marginalised and obliterated.

Chinese midwives, as a professional group, may not have been aware of these issues. Their profession was being victimised by the over-valuation of 'technology' and the devaluation of the human aspects of knowledge. It may take some time for the realisation to dawn that the modernisation of maternity care that midwifery brings include personal choice, humane maternity services and professional diversity. Midwives are challenged by new circumstances and intellectual grand theories and meta-narratives like modernisation, globalisation and postmodernism.

Third, the development of Chinese midwifery indicates an urgent need for an updated policy of support from the state health authorities. Particular attention is needed to encourage midwife-led birthing centres, evidence-based practice and good quality maternity care to protect women's interests. At the same time a legislative framework is required to benefit childbearing women and the healthy development of midwifery.

The evidence of our study has shown that the decline of Chinese midwifery was accelerated by the pathological increase in caesareans, especially within the urban areas; which resulted from the country's fast economic growth and increased medicalisation. The Fortaleza conference, convened by the World Health Organization, found that a caesarean rate above 10% cannot be justified on health grounds (Beech 2008), meaning that 90% of women can give birth vaginally. Thus, what women need are midwives not obstetricians. More studies should be commissioned to investigate the role of midwives in society, to investigate why normal birth centres or home births cannot be made possible for women and how Chinese midwifery can be structured to accommodate the different needs of individual women.

The fourth theme scrutinises the impact of the Western medical model of health care on Chinese midwifery. Western practice being applied in China has resulted in intervention becoming fashionable as well as dependence on machines. These issues frequently prompt intellectual analysis, including historical inquiries. Their occurrence is useful for thinking about the nature of midwifery practice, human needs and their long-term and short-term goals. Interventions, fashion and dependence suggest preferences, which is simply to say these techniques are available and the 'technological imperative' demands that they are used. Such phenomena are difficult to define and do not occur in isolation and this book has explored the ways in which the broad context shapes the ideologies surrounding their use.

The formal midwifery system in China is complemented by the lay system drawing on family, community and a variety of alternative healers. Chinese maternity care, as in many countries, is largely influenced by culture and society.

The slow start of midwifery and the suppression of the medical system facilitated this. All these factors have to be borne in mind when assessing midwifery's development. These themes are believed to provide crucial insights into the roles of Chinese midwives; such insights, in turn, facilitate the understanding and provide resources that could be used to create an effective infrastructure for an efficient midwifery service

Issues encountered

Three major issues encountered in this study are professionalisation, modernisation and marginalisation of Chinese midwifery. We think that for midwifery to take its rightful place as an important aspect of health care, it is necessary to understand these issues. The current state of and issues relating to midwifery cannot be separated from its historical development; therefore, the understanding of history and tradition is integrated throughout this book. How to overcome the division of work and the achievement of professional cooperation are discussed in depth in Part II. These issues are not only for Chinese midwifery to address but also for those in the West.

In the Western world there tends to be a functional separation between care and cure activities in which, for example, occupational roles are clearly demarcated between obstetricians, midwives and obstetric nurses. The hierarchy of a hospital environment may deprive midwives of their job satisfaction. In China midwives exist out-with formal organisational structures, being neither properly organised nor recognised as an independent profession. A large part of an obstetrician's role is spent doing the work of a midwife, while a midwife is doing that of a nurse or doula. This senseless 'job-hopping' is a frustrating phenomenon in Chinese midwifery.

These disjointed features of the past and present of Chinese midwifery are examples of the misinterpretation of health policy makers of the modern world. They reject their traditional assumptions and the premises of their predecessors. The converging and diverging interpretation of Chinese midwifery development behind these discontinuities and transformations are, for us, topics of endless fascination.

An understanding of the history of Chinese midwives, their jobs and their training was shown to indicate the working relationships of maternity care in Chinese society. It is also shown to be important in the process of industrialisation, modernisation and globalisation of obstetric technology in providing important symbols for the evaluation of conduct and standards of Chinese health workers.

The findings have led us to recognise our obligation to approach the development of Chinese midwifery with caution. In the first place, as midwives, we are not professional historians and our knowledge of history is limited. Second, our approach to this study cannot yield a large quantity of data. Finally, our profession as midwives may distort our interpretation of the past. Thus, we cannot claim to approach the data with complete detachment or to draw up a totally objective balance sheet of them.

However, this study represents an instrument of communication, giving content and meaning to the public. It is for them a frame of reference for social action. It also offers, to an important degree, criteria of value in types of maternity services. Furthermore, it provides an invaluable and irreplaceable record of the development of Chinese midwifery.

Where does Chinese midwifery go from here?

The machine-oriented income-generation enterprise that Chinese midwifery has become cannot be allowed to continue. Midwifery should serve the needs of women, babies and families with compassion, appreciation, consideration, respect and reverence for nature and natural rhythms. Midwives should be recognised by governments, policy-makers and educational institutions as being autonomous practitioners in their own right. They are not something in between doctors and nurses, but they may need to cooperate with other disciplines in an emergency. Midwives should and will, with the support of state policy, have their own professional body, universal examination standards, a unified registration, a career ladder and an updated review system.

Globally, there is growing consensus among public health professionals that midwifery provides care by working closely with women, babies, families, obstetricians and other health workers (Renfrew et al. 2014). Midwives are the main carers for the healthy woman, newborn and family from preconception to family formation. They are in the best position to care for healthy childbearing women and to keep birth normal (ICM 2014). The important contributions midwives make around the world are acknowledged in the reports of the UNFPPA et al. (2011, 2014). They are mainly on three fronts: saving the lives of women and children, as advocates for women's rights and as guardians of normal childbirth. The International Confederation of Midwives (ICM) supports this by envisaging 'a world where every childbearing woman has access to a midwife's care for herself and her newborn (ICM 2012).

Foreseeing the post-2030 Agenda for sustainable development (UN 2015), we advance a vision of the midwifery workforce in an integrated maternity system, holding the key to go beyond 'safe motherhood'. It is not only a political vision but a solution for improving the interactions and outcomes of a health system. We can operationalise this vision to organise our systems and policies to sustain and protect health.

It is important to establish a framework that supports maternity care with midwives as primary service providers and with assured back-up of specialist services. Assigning responsibility to midwives rests, in the end, on the support of midwives themselves, for example drawing up a policy of what procedure it is considered acceptable within a given community. This will include appropriate supervision and mentoring as well as technical and resource support and will require innovative professional development programmes promoted by state and provincial governments.

The promotion of normal birth and midwifery is a part of an innovative movement. The argument here is that 'normal birth' is the essence of midwifery for which midwives organise their care and services. 'Normal birth' may sound simple, but it is unbelievably complex in theory and in practice. It cuts through all areas surrounding midwifery, from women's health to the problems of medicine and medical technology. It touches on family building, married life and neonatal care. It is a new boundary in the maternity services, sociology and anthropology of health. That there has been such controversy over the definition of the term *normal birth* demonstrates its complexity.

Defining the concept of 'normal birth' develops into a process of learning and understanding health, illness and culture. The controversy arises out of social and cultural changes. As we have changed our lifestyles in the processes of industrialisation and socialisation, we have changed our ideas about what is normal and abnormal. If we think that change is what is normal in our cosmos, then normality should be viewed as a dynamic concept; we should be thinking about a multi-definitional approach contextualised in space and time. If the idea of 'normal birth' conjures up theoretical questions about birth, then 'care' tests these questions in practice.

Normalising childbirth is a process of transition from medicalisation of childbirth to giving birth physiologically. In the course of this process, the roles and identity of Chinese midwives are important, contingent, multiple and constantly being renegotiated. They are associated with the development of ideas and the development of maternity services and the changes of tradition. The continuing existence of tradition has always been a counterpoint to modernisation. The decline of traditional practice is one trend which does seem irreversible and the reinvention of tradition by designing new rules will be another trend. These new midwifery rules will be organised bodies of general knowledge, informed by, for example, descriptive, analytical and theoretical sciences of midwifery, sociology and history. Such knowledge will also be relevant to the midwifery professional body, policy-makers and administrators.

Implications for practice

We have been taking a critical look at the development of Chinese midwifery, which is largely influenced by its culture and society and involves both the lay and the formal midwifery systems. The formal midwifery system is balanced by the lay system drawing on family and community and by a variety of complementary healers. At the same time, we also have to maintain a critical distance, in order to be as objective as possible so that we can put the data into perspective to enable the midwives' accounts in our book to make overall sense.

The stories of Chinese midwives and midwifery in history and presently provide a framework for the understanding of how childbirth has been facilitated by them in China. As maternity care has been changed greatly over the years, many carers hold onto older ideas relating to birthing or define their present position according to the important debates of the past. The rapid social changes and the development of science and technology have induced indifference to and led to the decline of Chinese midwifery and its displacement by obstetrics. The dismal story of the modern midwife leader (see Chapter 10) clearly demonstrates this.

In this book we have argued that normal birth is the essence of midwifery as a part of women's reproductive health throughout their lives. Most healthy women want to have a fulfilling and uneventful pregnancy and birth. This can be achieved, first, by recognising the varied options for midwifery education for midwives so as to deliver flexible models of midwifery practice to meet the identified needs of the community and, second, by providing flexible models of care locally supported by midwives and accessible allied health, medical and specialist services.

The popularity of the midwife-led model in the country provides first-hand testimony of what and how people and individual midwives think about Chinese midwifery. The collective and individual views in their social settings help us to locate similarities and differences in different cultural constructs and restore the meanings, changing ideas and the development of Chinese midwifery.

The community of Chinese midwives is emerging but fluid. The current presence of traditional birth attendants, traditional midwives, doulas, nurse-midwives and nurse-midwife-obstetricians are reminders that Chinese midwives are not making full use of the opportunities available to them. They should focus on making a difference to women's birth experience and help to ground their supportive care in science and in a rational world. If they, especially their leaders, do not, the obstetric model and its instruments will replace them and their profession, and obstetric technology will be guaranteed the upper hand over humanity. This understanding can bridge the gap between the expression of the identity of Chinese midwives and the focus of their current attention and action on their services.

Regardless of whatever, even rudimentary, form Chinese midwifery takes, it exists and will thrive on evidence-based practice, clinical audit, professional development of the midwives and the support from diversity in practice and government policy. To demonstrate this is the prime task of this book. Such proof is essential to policy-making and administration. If Chinese midwives and their profession are to survive in the form in which they exist in the Netherlands, the UK and New Zealand, they will be obliged to undertake professional activities, such as research, to establish their roles in maternity care. Then their profession will thrive on continuing professional education and the support of state policies.

This book has presented how Chinese midwifery has facilitated childbirth in China. It fills a gap which exists in our knowledge. It provides a case for international communities to learn what midwifery is in China and calls for strategic planning and political action on the part of all midwives; furthermore, we argue support of the government's policy to strive for healthy intellectual development of midwives, midwifery in China and elsewhere to make a difference by improving the health and well-being of the population. We believe that the evidence and debate in this book will challenge and intrigue readers and show the way for future research.

Timeline of Chinese history

BCE (Before Common Era) and CE (Common Era) are used in this Timeline instead of the more familiar BC and AD as more appropriate to a study in which Christianity makes only a late appearance.

Features	Dynasty	Period
Feudal Age	*huángdì, zhuānxū, dìkù, yáo, shùn* 黄帝、颛顼、帝喾、尧、舜	2600–2100 BCE
	Xià Dynasty 夏	2200–1700 BCE
	Shāng Kingdom 商	1700–1100 BCE
	Zhōu Period 周	1100–256 BCE
	Warring states period *Zhànguó shídài* 战国时代	475–220 BCE
First Empire	*Qín* Dynasty 秦	221–206 BCE
	Hàn Dynasty 汉	206 BCE–220 CE
First Partition	Three Kingdoms 三国	220–280 CE
	Jìn Dynasty 晋	265–420
	Northern and Southern Empires 南北朝	420–589
Second Empire	*Suí* Dynasty 隋	581–618
	Táng Dynasty 唐	618–907
Second Partition	Five Dynasties & 10 countries 五代十国	907–960
Third Empire	*Sòng* Dynasty 宋	960–1279
Third Partition	*Liáo* Dynasty 辽	907–1125
	Jīn Dynasty 金	1115–1234
Fourth Empire	*Yuán* (Mongol) Dynasty 元	1206–1368
	Míng Dynasty 明	1368–1644
	Qīng (Manchu) Dynasty 清	1636–1911
Republic China (in Taiwan since 1949)	Republic of China 中华民国	Since 1912
Communist China (Mainland)	People's Republic of China (PRoC) 中华人民共和国	Since 1949

Guide to Chinese words and pronunciations

The *Pīnyīn* system

The official Chinese language was alphabetised by European scholars in the 19th and 20th centuries. An alphabetic system, based on the European alphabet, for standard spoken Chinese (*pǔtōnghuà* or 'common speech' known as Mandarin in English), has been developed by mainland Chinese since the 1950s. This is known as the *Pīnyīn* (to spell the sound). The system has been widely and success-fully used in schools throughout mainland China today. This book uses *Pīnyīn* for Chinese words where they appear. Chinese character writing is used when these words first appear.

The tones

Original Chinese words are monosyllabic, consisting mostly of one or two con-sonants and a vowel or a diphthong, with some words ending in nasals. This has resulted in many homophones (words of the same sound but with different mean-ings). The problem is treated by applying tones to the same sound for different words, making Chinese a tonal language. There are four tones in Mandarin Chi-nese (some dialects may have fewer or more): level, rising, falling-and-rising, falling. In writing in the *pīnyīn* system, diacritics are used on the main vowel sound to indicate the tones, for example *bā* (eight), *bá* (to pull up), *bǎ* (target or to hold), *bà* (father, dam or to give up).

Chinese names

The *pīnyīn* system with tones is used in this book for transcribing Chinese names. The name of a Chinese person, like other languages, consists of two parts: a family name and a given name. The family name usually comes first, as an individual is considered less important than the honour of the family. Most family names have one Chinese character or, occasionally, two characters. As to the given names, they usually have either one or two characters, for example *Chén Zìmíng* (陈自明; ca. 1190–1270), the author of the first comprehensive book on Chinese maternity care. Therefore, a person's full name normally consists of two characters or three, but sometimes four or more.

A person is usually known and called by others according to the situation he or she is in. For example, people have their childhood name (小名、乳名), nickname (外号), school name (学名), book name (书名), given name (名), literary name (associated with the meaning of the name or morality of the person with the name especially in ancient time; 表字or 字), official name (官名), courtesy name (号) and other name (别名). This practice has been criticised and punished by the communists and has declined since 1949 in mainland China. People normally just use their school names from then on in public. In this book all Chinese names are spelled in *pīnyīn* with their tones indicated, except those names chosen by the individuals.

Chinese emperor's titles

A Chinese emperor had a family name/surname, a given name and other names like anyone else, but the other people were not allowed to call him by these names. If they did, they would be punished for contempt of the emperor. There are two most common ways of referring to an emperor for his subjects. They are (1) by his Empire's Name (帝号) or Temple Name (庙号) and (2) by the year-period of his reign (年号).

An example of this is that the last emperor of the *Qīng* dynasty. His temple name is *Qīngxùndì* (清逊帝), and therefore, he is referred to as *Qīngxùn* Emperor. He ruled in two periods, the first was between 1908 and 1917, known as *Xuāntŏng* (宣统), which was the year-period he adopted for his dynasty; the second period was known as *Kāngdé* (康德) (between 1934 and 1945) for his puppet empire in *Shěnyáng* under Japanese occupation. These names are used with his imperial title as *Xuāntŏngdì* (宣统帝 *Xuāntŏng* Emperor) and *Kāngdédì* (康德帝 *Kāngdé* Emperor).

Xuāntŏngdì's family name is *Aisin-Gioro* (Manchu language, meaning the 'gold' family, which established and ruled China's *Qīng* dynasty). The *pīnyīn* spelling of *Aisin-Gioro* is *Àixīn Juéluó* (爱新觉罗). His given name is *Pŭ Yí* (.溥仪), while his childhood name is *Wŭgé* (午格); literary name, *Yàozhī* (耀之); courtesy name, *Hàorán* (浩然); and English name, Henry. But many of these personal names were not known to his subjects or to lay people of present time

Two basic year markings

There are two basic year markings in Chinese history used in this book: the dynastic cycle and continuous number of year rather like the BCE (Before Common Era) or CE (Common Era). *Kāngdé* year here is the year of the reign, which started from 1933 when the last *Qīng* emperor established his new palace in *Shěnyáng*. Hence, to exchange *Kāngdé* year to CE is simply to use 1933 plus the year of the reign.

Chinese glossary

Chinese pīnyīn	Chinese characters	Meaning
Běijīng	北京	Capital of China
Biǎn Què	扁鹊	*Biǎn Què* is a famous ancient medicine-man, who was a manager of a hotel in Qiu County, *Héběi* Province in the middle of warring states period (468–221 BCE). He was very kind to a customer who was a medicine-man. In return for his hospitality this medicine-man/customer taught *Biǎn Què* medicine, which he found very interesting (Liang 1983).
chǎnpó	产婆	Delivery woman in the community, birth attendant or traditional midwife
Fùdàn	复旦大学	*Fùdàn* University (in Shanghai)
fùkē	妇科	Gynaecology
Guǎngdōng	广东省	One of the 22 provinces in China
Guǎngzhōu	广州	The capital of *Guǎngdōng* Province
Guō Qǐzhōng's	郭稽中	The author of *Chǎnyù Bǎoqìngfāng*《产育宝庆方》which was written in 1109. The book helped Chinese midwifery to distinguish itself from Chinese medicine and become an independent subject.
Hángzhōu	杭州	The capital of *Zhèjiāng province*
Hànkǒu	汉口	A city in central China
hùshì	护士	Nurse, a new term was created from *kānhù* in China in 1909 when the Nurses' Association of China was established
jiēshēngpó	接生婆	Birth attendant, or traditional midwife
jiēshēngyuán	接生员	A modern term for birth attendant
jiēshēng, jiēshēng, bù jiē yě shēng	接生，接生，不接也生	A child is born anyway even if there is no assistance
jíyī	疾医	Internal medicine
kānchǎn	看产	Delivery watcher, birth attendant or traditional midwife
kàng	炕	Brick bed in northern China
kǎnshēngrén	看生人	Birth watcher, birth attendant or traditional midwife
Lǐ Shízhēn	李时珍	*Lǐ Shízhēn* based his work《本草纲目》(*Běn cǎo Gāngmù*, 1578) on folk tradition and more than 800 different herbal medicine books through the ages. He recorded 1892 herbs, of which 374 were discovered by him during his field collection.
Midwife	助产士	Trained midwives who work only in the labour wards in China
mǒushì shōuxǐ	某氏收洗	Aunty So-and-So, birth attendant and housekeeper, birth attendant or traditional midwife
Níngxià	宁夏	*Huí* Autonomous Region, one of the five autonomous regions in China.

Chinese pīnyīn	Chinese characters	Meaning
nüyī	女医	Medicine-woman, literate and skilled birth attendant who was chosen to serve in the palace and/or in the government office in feudal China,
Nurse midwife	助产士	Trained nurses who work in labour wards
Obstetric nurses	产科护士	In China it refers to nurses working in the department of gynaecology, antenatal, postnatal wards and community
Peking	北京	It is the formerly romanised name used for *Běijīng* before the standardisation of *pīnyīn* was introduced in the 1950s.
Pǔài	普爱护士学校	The name of a nursing school in *Hànkǒu*
qì	气	*Qì* (air) is a hypothetical concept in the eye of modern science, which refers to air, blood and body fluids in the human body. *Qì* is believed to be experienced and recognised as something of all reality, which is an invisible, dynamic and cosmic unity of the material world. It has the inherent property of *yīn* and *yáng* to reflect the simple concept of the unity of opposites.
Qīngdǎo	青岛市	One of the main ports for foreign trade in China. The city had a population of 7,156,500 and 75,631 births in 2002 (Qīngdǎo Government Net 2006). It was a German colony until the end of the World War I and was then occupied by Japan until it was handed over to the Nationalist government in 1929.
sāncóng sìdé	三从四德	A woman's three obediences (to father before marriage, to husband after marriage, and to son after husband's death) and four virtues (morality, proper speech, modest manner and diligent work). These are the spiritual fetters imposed on women in feudal society.
sāngū liùpó	三姑六婆	The literal translation is 'the three aunties and six grannies'. Three aunties were Buddhist nuns, Taoist nuns and soothsayers. The six grannies were brokers, matchmakers, shaman-healers, female pimps, drug dealers and delivery women. This expression first appeared in 1368 in *Táo Zōngyí*'s 陶宗仪 '*Chuò Gēn Lù*辍耕录' 'Stopping Farming' (CEEC 1979; Lee 1999; Leung 2000).
sānjiào jiǔliú	三教九流	The three religions (Confucianism, Taoism and Buddhism) and the nine schools of thought (Confucians, Taoists, *Yinyang*, Legalists, Logicians, Mohists, Political Strategists, Eclectics and Agriculturists. It is a derogatory term to refer to people in various trades, which first appeared in Xú Kè 'Qīng kē lèi chāo.nóngshāng lèi' 徐珂《清稞类钞.农商类》 around 220–280 CE (CEEC 1979: 22).

(*Continued*)

Chinese pīnyīn	Chinese characters	Meaning
sānshíliù héng	三十六行	Thirty-six walks of life. *Xú Kè 'Qīng kē lèi chāo. nóngshāng lèi'* 徐珂《清稗类钞.农商类》, doubles it; it becomes 72(七十二行), ten times, 360 (三百六十行). They all have the same meaning, that is people in different trades or all walks of life (CEEC 1979: 19)
Shèngjīng Women's Hospital	盛京女子医院	*Shèngjīng* Hospital in *Shěnyáng*, northern China, was one of the missionary hospitals established in 1883 by a Scottish missionary Dr Dugald Christie. *Shèngjīng* Hospital of China Medical (2007), *Wáng* et al. 1983: 3286–9 王树楠，吴廷燮.
shōushōng lǎolao	收生姥姥	Traditional birth attendant
sìbù	四部	A library system with 'four divisions' was established by the scholars of the imperial government between the 3rd and 4th centuries. The 'four divisions' were extended to 'four imperial libraries' (*sìkù*) in the 7th century.
sìkù	四库	Four Imperial Libraries, which were developed from *sìbù*. The collection from private and public ownership had reached 79,218 volumes with 3,471 subjects of all times by 18th century. The Emperor then had those perceived valuable and orthodox ones copied and re-organised into so-called Four Imperial Libraries with All Books (*Sìkù Quánshū*; Yang 1967).
Sìkù Quánshū	四库全书	The Four Imperial Libraries with All Books was an attempt made by the Chinese Emperor in the 18th century to organise a nationwide collection of all books in Chinese history which were considered valuable and orthodox. The collection included books of all subjects of all times in Chinese history up to that time.
Sìchuān	四川省	A province in south-west of China
shíyī	食医	Diet therapy
shōushēngpó	收生婆	Birth attendant, traditional midwife
shōushēng zhīfù	收生之妇	Birth receiving woman, birth attendant or traditional midwife
shòuyī	兽医	Veterinary medicine
Sūn Sīmiǎo	孙思邈	*Sūn Sīmiǎo* was born in 581 and died in 682 in Tang dynasty. When he was young he suffered poor health, so he decided to study medicine to help him and others. He was able to diagnose and prescribe herbal medicine to his neighbours and friends when he was about 20 (Liang 1983; Lee 1999).
'tàiyīshǔ'	太医署	Chinese imperial medical school in *Táng* dynasty (618–907 CE)
'tàiyīyuàn'	太医院	Chinese imperial medical school in *Sòng* dynasty (960–1279 CE)

Chinese pīnyīn	Chinese characters	Meaning
'tàiyījú'	太医局	Chinese imperial medical school in *Yuán* (Mongol) dynasty (1206–1368 CE)
Tānjīn	天津	A metropolis in northern coastal mainland China
wéiyī	为医	Being a doctor to serve the royal family in the Imperial Palace.
wěnpó	稳婆	Skilled but not necessarily literate birth attendant who was chosen to serve in the government office in feudal China; Birth calming woman (mainly served officials), a formal term for *shōushēngpó* 收生婆（Hu 1922a, b: 170）
wǔxíng	五行	The Five Elements or Five Phases. It is a fivefold conceptual scheme that many traditional Chinese fields use to explain a wide array of phenomena, from cosmic cycles to the interaction between human body and environment. The "Five elements" are Metal (金 *jīn*), Wood （木 *mù*), Water (水 *shuǐ*), Fire (火 *huǒ*) and Earth (土 *tǔ*).
xiàdì zuòcáo	下地坐草	To give birth on grass. It means the birth needs very basic care or is unattended.
Xīān	西安	Formerly romanised as Sian, also known as Chang'an ([tʂʰǎn.án]; Chinese: 长安; *pīnyīn : Cháng'ān*) before the Ming dynasty, is the capital of *Shaanxi* Province, People's Republic of China
Xīān Jiāotōng University	西安交通大学	It is one of the multidisciplinary research universities in China.
Yang Chóngruì	杨崇瑞	The headmistress of the first biomedical Chinese midwifery school, in Beijing.
yángyī	疡医	Surgery
Yínchuān	银川	The capital of *Níngxià Huí* Autonomous Region
yīnyáng	阴阳	*Yīn* originally meant 'shady'and is associated with the phenomena of cold, winter, cloud, rain, darkness; it symbolises femininity and negativity. *Yáng* means 'sunny' and is associated with heat, summer and symbolises masculinity and positivity. The *yīnyáng* system is the most basic division of the cosmos in traditional thought. This dualism has operated with every entity.
yuèsăo	月嫂	A female postnatal home help or housekeeper to help the new mother in her first month after birth.
Yuèzǐ bămǔ	月子保姆	A domestic nurse for a woman after giving birth in the first month
Zăn Yǐn	昝殷	A medicine-man, the author of the first book on Chinese midwifery and women's diseases. His book's name is *Jīngxiàochǎnbǎo* 《经效产保》 which was published either in 847 or in 853.
Zhèjiāng	浙江省	An eastern coastal province of China
Shēnzhèn	深圳市	A major city in *Guǎngdōng* Province
Zhōngguó	中国	The name of China in Chinese, meaning the 'Central Nation' or the Middle Kingdom

(*Continued*)

Chinese pīnyīn	Chinese characters	Meaning
zhùchǎnshì	助产士	Delivery person (it can be used to address either female or male midwife)
zhuòpó	坐婆	Traditional midwife, literally means a woman sitting (at birth); birth attendant or traditional midwife
zuùcáo fēnmiǎn	坐草分娩	Labour and deliver baby on grass
zuùrǔ fēnmiǎn	坐蓐分娩	Labour and deliver baby on a straw mat in the woman's bed (*Hángzhōu* custom; Hu 1922a: 167)

Further Reading and Notes

Useful websites

The following list of key websites may be useful.

English-language websites

1 http://chnm.gmu.edu/worldhistorysources/ World history Matters
2 http://internationalmidwives.org/ International Confederation of Midwives
3 www.rcm.org.uk/subject/midwifery-history The Royal College of Midwives
4 www.rcm.org.uk/news-views-and-analysis/analysis/the-midwives-act-1902-an-historical-landmark
5 http://wellcomelibrary.org/search-the-catalogues/ The library at Wellcome Collection
6 https://sourcebooks.fordham.edu/index.asp Fordham University's Internet History Sourcebooks Project, which is a Collection of public domain and copy-permitted historical texts presented clearly for educational use;
7 http://historymatters.gmu.edu/ History Matters: The U.S. Survey Course on the Web
8 http://afe.easia.columbia.edu/song/ A site on the Song dynasty (960–1279) in China examines the economic and social history of 12th-century China as seen through a scroll painting.
9 http://afe.easia.columbia.edu/ Asia for Educators, an initiative of the Weatherhead East Asian Institute at Columbia University
10 http://historians.org/ The American Historical Association

Chinese-language websites

1 www.nlc.gov.cn/ National Library of China, National Digital Library (中国国家图书馆, 中国国家数字图书馆）
2 www.yearbook.cn/ China Yearbook Online中国年鉴网
3 www.nlc.cn/nmcb/ National Museum of Chinese Classic Books (中国国家典籍博物馆)

4 www.duxiu.com/ An academic website in China (读秀学术搜索). It offers full-text search for: books, periodicals, newspapers, dissertations and conference papers.

5 www.nhfpc.gov.cn/zwgk/tjxx1/ejflist.shtml Statistics information of the National Health and Family Planning Commission of the People's Republic of China (NHFPC) (中华人民共和国卫生和计划生育委员会）

6 www.nhfpc.gov.cn/zwgk/tjnj1/ejlist.shtml China Health Statistics Yearbook （中华人民共和国卫生和计划生育委员会卫生统计年鉴）

7 www.nhfpc.gov.cn/fys/zcwj2/new_zcwj.shtml NHFPC's website for policies of maternity and child health

8 www.cmcha.org/detail/14610318864643300000.html The website for Midwives Branch of Maternal and Child Health Care of China Association (中国妇幼保健协会助产士分会)

9 www.cnzcs.com A private business website called Chinese Midwives Website (中国助产士网站).

10 www.obgy.cn/ A website of Obstetrics and Gynaecology in China created by an obstetrician and supported by his colleagues (中国妇产科网)

11 www.difangzhi.cn/ China Local Records Net (中国方志网), a national official website which aims to encourage and promote the chronicles and culture of each province, city and county in the country

12 www.bjdfz.gov.cn/ *Běijīng* Geographical Information Network (北京地情资料网)

13 www.tjdfz.org.cn/tjtz/wsz/dashijilve/index.shtml *Tiānjīn* Local Chronicles: *Tiānjīn*>Health天津地方志网：天津通志>卫生志

14 www.shtong.gov.cn/newsite/node2/index.html *Shànghǎi* Local Chronicles 上海市地方志办公室

15 www.fjsq.gov.cn/ Local Chronicles Compilation Committee of *Fújiàn* Province (福建省地方志编纂委员会)

16 www.hangzhou.gov.cn/col/col805745/index.html *Hángzhōu* Chronicles (杭州市志)

Traditional Chinese medicine books pertinent to midwifery

(A chronological list)

Timeline	Features
Dōng Zhōu dynasty东周 (770–256 BCE)	*Huángdì-nèijīng* (*The Yellow Emperor's Book of Medicine* 《黄帝内经》) was believed to be written in this period (Jia 1982; Liang 1983; Furth 1999). It is a collected work and consists of two sections: *Sùwèn* 《素问》 and *Língshū* 《灵枢》. www.gushiwen.org/guwen/huanglei.aspx (Last accessed 18 Aug 2017).
Hàn 汉 (206 BCE–220 CE)	*Sùnǚfang bufenjuan*《素女方不分卷》, Unknown author www.tsg.ynutcm.edu.cn/szzy/sysjk/15990.shtml (Last accessed 21 Aug 2017).
Táng 唐 (618–907 CE) 652	*Bèijí-qiānjīn yàofāng* 《备急千金要方》30 chapters, *Sūn Sīmiǎo* (孙思邈) (ed) in 652 CE (Fu et al. 1982; Liang 1983). It is also known as *qiānjīn yàofāng*《千金要方》. http://zhongyibaodian.com/archives/15123.html (Last accessed 19 Aug 2017).
	Qiānjīn bǎoyào《千金宝要》6 vols, *Sūn Sīmiǎo* (孙思邈) (ed) http://zhongyibaodian.com/qianjinbaoyao/ (Last accessed 21 Aug 2017)
682 (Fu et al. 1982)	*Qiānjīn yìfāng*《千金翼方》30Vols, *Sūn Sīmiǎo* (孙思邈). *Sūn*'s two books were *Bèijí-qiānjīn yàofāng* 《备急千金要方》(652AD) *Qiānjīn yìfāng*《千金翼方》(682 CE) were also known as *Qiānjīnfāng*, 《千金方》. http://zhongyibaodian.com/qianjinyifang/ (Last accessed 19 Aug 2017).
752	《外台秘要》*Wàitāi mìyào* 40vols, 1104 subjects *Wáng Tāo* (王涛) (670–755) http://zhongyibaodian.com/archives/15655.html (Last accessed 21 Aug 2017).
762	*Huángdì-nèijīng-sùwèn* 《黄帝内经素问》(*Questions on Yellow Emperor's Book of Medicine*) (*Wáng* 762, Liang 1983). www.tcm100.com/user/hdnjsw/index.htm http://ishare.iask.sina.com.cn/f/ouPIq6USoG.html (Last accessed 19 Aug 2017).
847 or 853	*Jīng-xiào-chǎn-bǎo*《经效产宝》, *Zǎn Yǐn* (昝殷). This is the first book on Chinese midwifery and gynaecology. www.wenkuxiazai.com/doc/932936166529647d272852ba.html (Last accessed 19 Aug 2017).
Sòng 宋 (960–1279)	
1098年	*Shíchǎn Lùn*《十产论》, *Yáng Zǐjiàn* (杨子建). http://zhongyibaodian.com/jiyingangmu/614-18-6.html (Last accessed 19 Aug 2017).
1109	*Chǎn-yù-bǎo-qìng-fāng* 《产育宝庆方》, *Guō Qǐzhōng* (郭稽中) separated midwifery from Chinese medicine in his book in Song dynasty, and midwifery became an independent subject since then. http://ishare.iask.sina.com.cn/f/24742163.html (Last accessed 20 Aug 2017).
1127	*Chǎnyù bǎojīng*《产育宝经》(Li et al. 1127).

(Continued)

Timeline	Features
1184	*Wèishēng jiabǎo chǎnkē bèiyào*《卫生家宝产科备要》8 Vols, *Zhū Duānzhāng*朱端章. http://zhongyibaodian.com/weishengjiabaochankebeiyao5682/ (Last accessed 20 Aug 2017).
1220	*Nǔkē bǎiwèn*《女科百问》2 Vols, *Qí Zhòngfǔ* (齐仲甫) (Qi 1983) http://zhongyibaodian.com/nvkebaiwen/ (Last accessed 20 Aug 2017).
	Chǎnbǎo zhùfāng《产宝諸方》1 Vol, Unknown author. www.doc88.com/p-6901156522147.html (35 pages) (Last accessed 20 Aug 2017).
1237	*Fùrén dàquán Liáng fāng*《妇人大全良方》24 Vols, *Sòn-jiā-xī-yuánián, Chén Zì-míng* (陈自明) (ca. 1190–1270) (Chen 1237; Fu et al. 1982, Liang 1983; Leung 2000). It is the first comprehensive book on Chinese midwifery and gynaecology. http://zhongyibaodian.com/furendaquanliangfang/ (Last accessed 20 Aug 2017).
Yuán 元 (1206–1368)	*Gézhìyúlún*《格致余论》by *Zhū Zhèhēn* (朱震亨) (1281–1358). A monograph (41 chapters) of the author's understanding about Chinese medicine, surgery, women's and children's diseases and the care of the elderly. www.baike.com/wiki/%25E3%2580%258A格致余论%25E3%2580%258B#1 (Last accessed 30 Aug 2017).
Míng 明 (1368–1644)	*Nǔkē cuōyào*《女科撮要》2 Vol, *Xuē Yǐ* (薛已) (Book Library 2005). http://zhongyibaodian.com/nvkecuoyao/ (Last accessed 16 Apr 2018).
1425	*Fùqīngzhǔ nǔkē*《傅青主女科》2 Vols (Fu 1425), *Fù Shān* (傅山) (ca. 1607–1685) (published in1827) (Fu 1425a, b, Liang 1983, Furth 1987). http://zhongyibaodian.com/fuqingzhunvke5190/ (Last accessed 20 Aug 2017.
1531	*History of Chinese Medicine*《医学正传》Yu, T. (虞抟). (reprinted in 1965). People's Health Publishing House, Běijīng.
?1596	*Yìnchǎn quánshū*《胤产全書》4 Vols, *Wáng Kěntáng* (王肯堂).
1549	*Wànshì nǔkē*《万氏女科》3 Vols. http://zhongyaofangji.com/book/wanshinvke-565.html (Last accessed 20 Aug 2017).
	Wànshì jiāchuán nǔkē yàoyán《万氏家传女科要言》4 Vols, *Wàn Quán* (万全) (ca. 1488–1580).
	Fùrén guī《妇人规》2 vol. *Zhāng Jièbīn* (张介宾) http://zhongyibaodian.com/furengui/ (Last accessed 21 Aug 2017).
Qīng 清 (1616–1911)	
1715	*Dá shēng piān*《达生篇》(On successful childbirth) 亟斋居士*Jí zhāi jū-shì* (Furth 1987). https://zhongyibaike.com/wiki/%E8%BE%BE%E7%94%9F%E7%AF%87 (Last accessed 20 Aug 2017).

Timeline	Features
1716	*Gōng Tíngxian* (龚廷贤) *Nèifŭ mìchuán nŭkē*《内府秘传经验女科》 http://zhongyibaodian.com/neifumichuanjingyannvke5355/ (Last accessed 21 Aug 2017).
1731	*Tāichăn xīnfă*《胎产心法》3 Vols, *Yán Cún-xĭ* (阎纯玺). http://zhongyibaodian.com/taichanxinfa/ (Last accessed 20 Aug 2017).
1736–1796	*Fùkē yùchĭ*《妇科玉尺》6 Vols, *Shĕn Jīnáo* (沈金鳌). http://zhongyibaodian.com/fukeyuchi/ (Last accessed 20 Aug 2017).
1781	*Tāichăn jíyào*《胎产集要》(*Essentials of pregnancy and childbirth*), *Huáng Tì-zhāi* (黄惕齋) http://book.kongfz.com/item_pic_13255_632530119/ (Last accessed 20 Aug 2017).
1782	*Nŭkē Jīnlún*《女科经纶》8 Vols, Xiāo Xūn (萧埙). http://zhongyibaodian.com/nvkejinglun/670-5-1.html (Last accessed 20 Aug 2017).
1786	*Zhúlínsìnŭkē*《竹林寺女科》(*Medical care for women from the Bamboo Forest Temple*), The monks in the Bamboo Forest Temple竹林寺僧 (Furth 1987) *Zhúlín nŭkē zhèngzhì*《竹林女科证治》4 vols http://zhongyibaodian.com/zhulinnvkezhengzhi/ (Last accessed 21 Aug 2017).
1795	*Tāichăn mìshū*《胎产秘书》（*Secrets of pregnancy and childbirth*）*Chén Hùān* (陈笏庵) (Furth 1987) http://ishare.iask.sina.com.cn/f/22931027.html (37 pages); http://zhongyibaodian.com/taichanmishu5698/ (Last accessed 20 Aug 2017).
1827	*Fùqīngzhŭ nŭkē*《傅青主女科》2 Vols & 2 postnatal Vols attached, *Fù Shān* (傅山). Written in Ming Dynasty. http://zhongyibaodian.com/archives/22986.html (Last accessed 20 Aug 2017).
1830	*Chăn-yùn-jí*《产孕集》(14 chapters) *Zhāng Zhòng-yuăn,* (张仲远). http://yuedu.163.com/source/e17613bbafc84847954e8988bd97a0bd_4 (Last accessed 20 Aug 2017).
1862	*Nŭkē jíyào*《女科辑要》Other name: *Shĕnshì Nŭkē jíyào*《沈氏女科辑要》2 Vols, *Shĕn Yòu-péng* (沈又彭). http://ishare.iask.sina.com.cn/f/9759261.html (29 pages) (Last accessed 20 Aug 2017). www.guoxuedashi.com/a/9175j/75851f.html (Last accessed 21 Aug 2017).
1877	*Nŭkē yāo lüĕ*《女科要略》*Pān Wèi* (潘蔚) (1816–1894). The book consists of care & treatment provided in 4 sections: menstruation, threatened miscarriage, birth and postpartum period. www.baike.com/wiki/%E3%80%8A%E5%A5%B3%E7%A7%91%E8%A6%81%E7%95%A5%E3%80%8B (Last accessed 20 Aug 2017).《女科精要》3 vols. Unknown author, Unknown year of publication. http://zhongyibaodian.com/nvkejingyao/ (Last accessed 21 Aug 2017).

Midwifery policies in China

Table 3.1 Midwifery policies of the Nationalist government of China, 1911–1949 (17 policies, chronologically)

Date of publication	Policy	Departments of Publication	Sources
1913	The provisional ban of birth attendants issued by the Department of Capital Police of *Běiyáng* government 《京师警察厅暂行取缔产婆规则》	Department of the Capital's Police of *Běiyáng* Government (1912–28) of the Republic of China (1911-date)北洋政府京师警察厅	Cai H 1999 ed. Collection of the *Regislations of the republic of China. Vol 26.* Huangshan Publishing Society, Hefei: 69–70. 蔡鸿源主编：《民国法规集成》合肥黄山书社第26册，第69–70页www.iolaw.org.cn/showNews.aspx?id=51601 (Last accessed 3 Apr 2017).
1928	Regulations governing the registration of midwives 管理助产女士（产婆）暂行章程	Municipality of Greater Shanghai上海特别市市政府卫生局	It contains 28 articles, doubles that of the Midwives Rules.
9 Jul 1928 Amended 21 May 1929	Chinese Midwives Rules 《助产士条例》	Ministry of Health, Republic of China民国卫生部	Chinese Ministry of Health. www.jkcsw.com/hlzt/hlgl/200601/15259.html. (Last accessed 7 Jun 2008). http://book.xuexi365.com/ebook/detail.jhtml?id=10817564&page=4 (Last accessed 30 Mar 2017): 79–81/356
31 Jul 1928 Amended 22 Jun 1939	Management Rules for Birth Attendants 《管理接生婆规则》	Ministry of the Interior内政部	http://book.xuexi365.com/ebook/detail.jhtml?id=10817564&page=4 (Last accessed 30 Mar 2017): 27–9/356
30 Jan 1929 Amended 16 Jun 1937	Rules of Midwifery Educational Board 《助产教育委员会章程》	Ministry of Education & Ministry of the Interior	Department of Compiling Committee. 1936. *Almanac of the health.* 4th ed. The Commercial Press: 302–3. 《民国医药卫生法规选编（1912–1948）》http://book.xuexi365.com/ebook/detail.jhtml?id=10817564&page=4 (Last accessed 9 Apr 2017): 237/356
13 Mar 1929	Rules of Midwives' Examination 助产士考试规则	Ministry of Health	Chen MG. 1996.*The Historical Selection of Chinese Health Legislations: 1912 to 1949.* The Press of *Shanghǎi* Medical University. Shanghai: 743
Dec 1929	Regulation of Setting up Training Class for Birth Attendants	Ministry of Health	Chen MG. 1996. *The Historical Selection of Chinese Health Legislations: 1912 to 1949.* The Press of *Shanghǎi* Medical University. shanghai: 746–7

Date	Title	Issuing body	Source
3 Apr, 1931	Rules of Special Examination for Midwives 《特种考试助产士考试条例》	Ministry of Health	《民国医药卫生法规选编（1912–1948）》http://book.xuexi365.com/ebook/detail.jhtml?id=10817564&page=4 (Last accessed 30 Mar 2017):139–140/356
16 Jun, 1931	Revised Standard of Educational System and Courses on Midwifery School	Midwifery Educational Committee	Chen MG. 1996. *The Historical Selection of Chinese Health Legislations: 1912 to 1949.* The Press of *Shànghǎi* Medical University. shanghai: 722
25 Feb, 1937	Rules of Setting up Special Midwifery Class in Advanced Midwifery Vocational School	Ministry of Education	Chinese Ministry of Education. The newly news of vocational education. *Occupation and Education.* 1937, 148: 342–3
16 Jun 1937 amended Rules set on 30 Jan 1929	Amended rules of the Midwifery Education Board 《修正助产教育委员会章程》	Ministry of Education, Ministry of the Interior 民国教育部内政部	《民国医药卫生法规选编（1912–1948）》http://book.xuexi365.com/ebook/detail.jhtml?id=10817564&page=4 (Last accessed 30 Mar 2017): 237–8/356
22 Jun 1939	Amended Rules for Birth Attendants 《修正管理接生婆规则》	Ministry of the Interior 民国内政部	《民国医药卫生法规选编（1912–1948）》http://book.xuexi365.com/ebook/detail.jhtml?id=10817564&page=4 (Last accessed 30 Mar 2017): 239–241/356
8 Aug 1940	Interim Regulations on Midwives 《助产士暂行条例》	State Council 民国行政院	《民国医药卫生法规选编（1912–1948）》http://book.xuexi365.com/ebook/detail.jhtml?id=10817564&page=4 (Last accessed 30 Mar 2017): 265–6/356
30 Sep 1943	Midwives Rules (Amended) 《助产土法》 (including the regulations of midwives associations)	Nationalist Government 民国国民政府	Archives of *Zhèjiāng* Province: L029–004–0232 Nationalist Government. www.med66.com/html/ziliao/07/89/e9ac1f73be8c01643159351 4e9d70ea1.htm (Last accessed 31 Mar 2017). 《民国医药卫生法规选编（1912–1948）》http://book.xuexi365.com/ebook/detail.jhtml?id=10817564&page=4 (Last accessed 30 Mar 2017): 293–7/356

(Continued)

Table 3.1 (Continued)

Date of publication	Policy	Departments of Publication	Sources
8 Jul 1944	Regulations for Checking Medical Practitioners, Pharmacists and Midwives《医师、药剂师及助产士检覆办法》	Chinese Examination Board, Chinese Political Board	Archives of *Zhèjiāng* Province: L029–004–0233 *Chóngqìng* Archives: 0053–2–1169
21 Jul 1945	Rules for the Implement of Medical Practitioners《医师法施行细则》	Ministry of Health 民国卫生署	*Hángzhōu* Archives: L008–002–063 《民国医药卫生法规选编（1912–1948）》http:/book.xuexi365.com/ebook/detail.jhtml?id=10817564&page=4 (Last accessed 30 Mar 2017): 302–3/356
21 Jul 1945	Midwives Act Enforcement Rules《助产士法施行细则》	Ministry of Social Affairs, Ministry of Health 民国社会部，卫生署会	《民国医药卫生法规选编（1912–1948）》http:/book.xuexi365.com/ebook/detail.jhtml?id=10817564&page=4 (Last accessed 30 Mar 2017): 306–7/356

Table 3.2 Maternity care policies of the People's Republic of China, 1950–2017 (63 policies, chronologically)

	Date	Policy	Department	Sources	Interpretation
1.	4 Apr, 1951	Provincial rules for the management of hospitals & clinics 医院诊所管理暂行条例	State Council (SC)	http://www.gov.cn/banshi/2005-08/01/content_19113.htm (Last accessed 10 Apr 2017).	Revoked on 1 Sep 1994
2.	24 Apr, 1952	Temporary Regulations of Medical Assistants, Assistant Pharmacists, Nurses and Midwives.	Ministry of Health of the (MoH)	Chinese Ministry of Health. http://www.jkcsw.com/hlzt/hlgl/200601/15266.html/ (Last accessed 10 Mar 2008).	There were five categories: medicine, public health, pharmacy, laboratory and others. Midwives were classified as intermediate level skill workers.
3.	Apr, 1956	National health workers' job titles and job promotion Ordinance (draft)" 国家卫生技术人员职务名称和职务晋升暂行条例 (草案)	MoH	Zhèjiāng Archive J165-006-013	This bill was amended in May 1963 by the CMoH. No job promotion 1966-1970
4.	2 Dec, 1978	The principles for the organization of a General Hospital (draft) 综合医院组织编制原则 (试行草案)	MoH	http://www.law-lib.com/law/law_view.asp?id=1882 (Last accessed 14 Jul 2012).	Hospital staffing: 1bed:1.3-7 staff; 1 doctor: 1 nurse. 'Midwife' was mentioned five times in the document. It was included under 'nurses'.
5.	23 Feb, 1979	The Regulations of Health Workers' Duty and Promotion (For Trial Implementation)	MoH	Chinese Ministry of Health. http://192.168.209.242/elaw (Last accessed 18 Mar 2008).	
6.	15 Jun, 1980	Maternal & child health care (Trial) 妇幼卫生工作条例 (试行草案)	MoH	http://www.law-lib.com/Law/law_view.asp?id=313374 (Last accessed 30 Mar 2017).	Details the hierarchy, structures, functions & ratio of maternity care system. Doctors are the main workforce, midwives, barefoot doctors & birth attendants also mentioned
7.	11 Feb, 1983	Working conference of the National Maternal and Child Health 《全国妇幼卫生工作会议纪要》国务院办公厅国办发 [1983] 12号颁布	SC	http://vip.chinalawinfo.com/Newlaw2002/SLC/slc.asp?gid=1548 (Last accessed 30 Mar 2017).	This is the first of its kind. Midwifery schools and midwifery training were suggested to tackle the acute shortage of maternity care workers and to overcome the monopoly of state run hospitals

(Continued)

Table 3.2 (Continued)

	Date	Policy	Department	Sources	Interpretation
8.	1 Jun, 1985	The standards and requirements of the quality of maternal health services in urban and rural areas 全国城乡孕产期保健质量标准和要求	MoH	http://www.law-lib.com/law/law_view.asp?id=3207 (Last accessed 14 Jul 2012).	Revoked on 23 Jun 2011
9.	30 Jun, 1986	The principles of the organisation of an Obstetric and gynecology hospital (Trial) 妇产科专科医院组织编制原则 （试行）	MoH	http://law.51labour.com/lawshow-43207-2.html (Last accessed 14 Jul 2017).	Revoked on 23 Jun 2011 No mention of 'midwife' but 'nursing staff' (护理人员), which comprised nurses and doctors. Labour was perceived as two stages: pre-labour and labour periods in terms of staff management. Bed & staff ratio: 1:1-1.7; Bed & outpatient number: 1:2-2.5. These ratios have never been realised clinically.
10.	20 Apr, 1987	National Urban Perinatal Care Management (Trial) 全国城市围产保健管理办法 （试行）	MoH	http://www.law-lib.com/lawhtm/1987/4245.htm (Last accessed 23 Nov 2017).	Revoked on 23 Jun 2011 Midwife was mentioned once. Her job was defined as making records and reports.
11.	10 Feb, 1989a	Rural maternal health Management (Trial) 农村孕产妇系统保健管理办法 （试行）	MoH	法律网《法律法规查询《行政法类《医药卫生＜母婴保健 http://www.chinalawedu.com/news/1200/22598/22621/22908/2006/5/li7443164147122560021 7020-0.htm (Last accessed 21 Aug 2017).	Revoked on 23 Jun 2011 1. Rural perinatal check-ups were started from 12 weeks 2. Antenatal booking, visits & post-natal visits were clearly described, but no clear description about labour and delivery process. 3. Newborns skin-to-skin contact was mentioned.
12.	10 Feb, 1989b.	The routine of a home delivery (Trial) 家庭接生常规 （试行）	MoH	http://www.law-lib.com/law/law_view.asp?id=50202 (Last accessed 30 Mar 2017).	Revoked on 23 Jun 2011 Acknowledged home birth predominates in rural and remote areas. Details equipment, procedures, recordings, requirements and indications for transfer, dos & don'ts especially. 3 stages of labour.

No.	Date	Title	Body	URL	Description
13.	10 Feb, 1989c	Regulation for rural birth attendants (trial) 农村助产人员管理条例(试行)	MoH	http://www.law-lib.com/law/law_view.asp?id=5533 (Last accessed 30 Mar 2017).	Revoked on 23 Jun 2011 Carers consist of village doctor, health workers, birth attendants, traditional midwives
14.	22 Jan, 1992	The standards for the development of a maternity hospital 妇幼保健院、所建设标准（报批稿）	MoH	http://wenku.baidu.com/view/4cb318ec5ef7ba0d4a733b26.html (Last accessed 21 Aug 2017).	It is mainly about the environment, equipment, size of floor areas and building allocation of the clinical, paramedical and management areas
15.	26 Feb 1994a	Management regulations of medical institutions 医疗机构管理条例	SC	http://www.gov.cn/banshi/2005-08/01/content_19113.htm (Last accessed 10 Apr 2017).	Replaced the 1951 version Hospital with <100 beds needs to apply local government & review registration annually; > 100 beds, provincial government, review every 3 yrs.
16.	27 Oct, 1994b	Maternal and Child Health Law of the People's Republic of China 中华人民共和国母婴保健法	MoH	http://www.moh.gov.cn/publicfiles/business/htmlfiles/mohzcfgs/s3576/200804/17584.htm (Last accessed 21 Aug 2017).	Requires urban people by law to have a health check-up before marriage registration; but does not apply to rural and remote areas because of the financial difficulties.
17.	7 Aug, 1995a	The management methods for the licence and qualification of maternal and child health services 母婴保健专项技术服务许可及人员资格管理办法	MoH	http://www.moh.gov.cn/publicfiles/business/htmlfiles/mohfybjysqwss/s7899/200804/17614.htm (Last accessed 21 Aug 2017).	A total of 20 articles including health check-ups, sterilisation, artificial abortion, licensing, audits and so on.
18.	7 Aug, 1995b	Basic standard of maternal and child healthcare services 母婴保健专项技术服务基本标准	MoH	http://www.moh.gov.cn/publicfiles/business/htmlfiles/mohfybjysqwss/s7900/200804/17615.htm (Last accessed 21 Aug 2017).	The regulations and requirements in 3 areas: 1. Medical check-ups before marriage registration; 2. Termination of pregnancy; 3. Basic standard for home delivery.
19.	7 Aug, 1995c	The appraisal of maternal and child health medical technologies 母婴保健医学技术鉴定管理办法	MoH	http://www.moh.gov.cn/publicfiles/business/htmlfiles/mohfybjysqwss/s7899/200804/17616.htm (Last accessed 21 Aug 2017).	The appraisal committee consists of five experts from different disciplines in medical technologies.

(Continued)

Table 3.2 (Continued)

	Date	Policy	Department	Sources	Interpretation
20.	15 Jan, 1999	The Standards of Professional Structure of Secondary Medical Education	MoH, & Ministry of Education (MoE)	Ministry of Health, Ministry of Education. http://192.168.209.242/elaw/ApiSearch.dll?ShowRecordText?Db=chl&Id=0&Gid=65189&ShowLink=false&PreSelectId=2894905536&Page=0&PageSize=20#m_font_0 (Last accessed 3 Mar 2008). www.moh.gov.cn	
21.	20 Feb, 2001	Management of human assisted reproductive technology 人类辅助生殖技术管理办法	MoH	www.moh.gov.cn	Five chapters with 25 articles. The focus is on artificial insemination, in vitro fertilization and its various derivative technologies
22.	30 Apr, 2001	The Extensive Planning about Responsibility System of Continuous Midwifery care in the Labour Unit in *Shēnzhèn*	Health Bureau of *Shēnzhèn*	Health Bureau of *Shēnzhèn*. http://www.fsou.com/html/text/lar/169590/16959032.html. (Last accessed 2 Oct 2008).	
23.	20 Jun, 2001	The implementation measures of the maternal and Child Health Law of the People's Republic of China 中华人民共和国母婴保健法实施办法 (第308号)	MoH	http://www.moh.gov.cn/publicfiles/business/htmlfiles/mohzcfgs/s3576/200804/29521.htm (Last accessed 23 Nov 2017).	Eight chapters with 45 articles. 'Informed choice' for the first time found its way into the document, but there has not been much research evidence for women
24.	29 Dec, 2001	Population and family law of the People's Republic of China 中华人民共和国人口与计划生育法 (中华人民共和国主席令第63号)	MoH	http://www.moh.gov.cn/mohzcfgs/pzcfg/list_6.shtml Accessed 31 Mar 2017	Seven chapters with 47 articles.
25.	17 Jun, 2002	The Standard of Premarital Health Care (Amended) 婚前保健工作规范〈修订〉(147号)	MoH	http://www.gov.cn/banshi/2005-08/23/content_25506.htm (Last accessed 23 Nov 2017).	Four sections comprising a simplified version of the document of 17 Jun 2002.

No.	Date	Title	Agency	URL	Notes
26.	Aug, 2002	Baby Friendly Hospital Management Guide 爱婴医院管理监督指南	Division of Maternal and Child Health, MoH	http://www.moh.gov.cn/mohfybjysqwss/s6746/200804/18200.shtml (Last accessed 23 Nov 2017).	Just a list of items.
27.	4 Apr, 2002	Regulations of Medical Malpractice 医疗事故处理条例 (国务院令第351号)	SC	http://www.gov.cn/banshi/2005-08/02/content_19167.htm (Last accessed 23 Nov 2017).	63 articles taking effect on 1 Sep 2002.
28.	24 Sep, 2002	Administrative measures for antenatal diagnostic techniques 产前诊断技术管理办法(第33号) Implemented 1 May 2003	MoH	http://www.law-lib.com/law/law_view.asp?id=42544 (Accessed 31 Mar 2017)	Antenatal diagnostic tests were widely used clinically for reassurance or family planning rather than to assess fetal well-being.
29.	12 Feb, 2004	Guide to a baby friendly hospital management 爱婴医院管理监督指南	MoH	http://www.moh.gov.cn/mohfybjysqwss/s6746/200804/18200.shtm (Last accessed 23 Nov 2017).	Mixed feeding with milk or sugary water before mother's milk comes in is still a popular and acceptable in Chinese hospitals.
30.	24 May, 2004	The Planning of Developing and Reforming Higher Education of Nursing, Pharmacy and Other Medical Relevant Professions	MoH & MoE	Chinese Ministry of Health, Chinese Ministry of Education. http://192.168.209.242/elaw (Last accessed 23 Nov 2017).	
31.	23 Jun, 2004	Notice of free pre-marital health advice and guidance announced by Ministry of Health 卫生部关于免费开展婚前保健咨询和指导的通知	MoH	http://www.moh.gov.cn/mohbgt/pw10407/200804/27025.shtml (Last accessed 21 Aug 2017).	The departments of health at all levels were advised by the MoH to provide premarital health services & guidelines to women and men free of charge for medical institutions.
32.	27 Dec, 2004	Specifications of the neonatal screening technology 《新生儿疾病筛查技术规范》	MoH	http://www.moh.gov.cn/publicfiles/business/htmlfiles/mohfybjysqwss/s6746/200804/18192.htm (Last accessed 22 Aug 2017).	
33.	31 Mar, 2005	The approval of the Ministry of Health on the disposal of placenta 卫生部关于产妇分娩后胎盘处理问题的批复	MoH	http://www.moh.gov.cn/publicfiles/business/htmlfiles/mohzcfgs/s6730/200804/29741.htm (Last accessed 21 Aug 2017).	Placenta is the property of the mother. ○ Placental trading is banned.

(Continued)

Table 3.2 (Continued)

	Date	Policy	Department	Sources	Interpretation
34.	19 Dec, 2006	The Ministry of Health on the issuance of the notice of the maternal and child health institutions management approach 卫生部关于印发《妇幼保健机构管理办法》的通知(卫妇社发[2006]489)	MoH	http://www.moh.gov.cn/mohfybjysqwss/s6746/200804/18804.shtml (Last accessed 21 Aug 2017).	There are eight chapters. Many rules were set up, but not many have been described clearly and implementable, for example, the ratio between clinician and beds were: 1:1.7
35.	22 Dec, 2006	The MoH guidance for strengthening maternal and child health 卫生部关于进一步加强妇幼卫生工作的指导意见 卫妇社发[2006]495号	MoH	http://www.gov.cn/gzdt/2007-01/05/content_488355.htm (Last accessed 21 Aug_2017).	Full of empty big words unrelated to specifics.
36.	5 Jan, 2007	《妇幼保健机构管理办法》	MoH	http://www.moh.gov.cn/publicfiles/business/htmlfiles/mohfybjysqwss/s6746/200804/18186.htm (Last accessed 21 Aug 2017).	
37.	26 Feb, 2007	Preconception care services (Trial) 《孕前保健服务工作规范（试行）》[卫妇社发（2007)56号]	MoH	http://www.moh.gov.cn/publicfiles/business/htmlfiles/mohfybjysqwss/s6746/200804/18185.htm (Last accessed 21 Aug 2017).	Institutionalized antenatal care,
38.	11 Jan, 2008	The public directory and texts of maternal and child health institutions (Draft)" 《妇幼保健机构信息公开目录和规范文本（征求意见稿）》(卫妇社卫卫便函[2008]5号)	MoH	http://www.moh.gov.cn/publicfiles/business/htmlfiles/mohfybjysqwss/s7901/200804/18184.htm (Last accessed 21 Aug 2017)	Tabulation of information to put up posters and send messages to the media and hospitals
39.	23 Jan, 2008	Nurses Ordinance 《护士条例》	SC & MoH	http://www.gov.cn/zwgk/2008-02/04/content_882178.htm (Last accessed 23 Nov 2017).	This is the first law for nurses in China since 1949. It has 35 articles. The term midwife is mentioned once. It was confined to midwifery courses at college level.

#	Date	Title		URL	Notes
40.	4 May, 2008	Method for the registration of Nurse practitioners 护士执业注册管理办法	MoH	http://www.gov.cn/flfg/2008-05/12/content_968012.htm (Last accessed 21 Aug 2017).	The term midwife is mentioned once. It was confined to midwifery courses at college level.
41.	23 Jun, 2008	Notice of the activities of the 2008 World Breastfeeding Week 2008年"世界母乳喂养周"活动的通知[卫办妇社发〔2008〕123号]	MoH	http://www.moh.gov.cn/mohfybjsqwss/s3586/200807/37130.shtml (Last accessed 21 Aug 2017).	Staff and health institutions at all levels are banned from selling milk substitutes to the family of pregnant women for profit.
42.	21 Jul, 2008	Post-disaster emergency program of maternal and child health services 《灾后妇幼卫生服务应急方案》卫办妇社发〔208〕37号	MoH	http://www.moh.gov.cn/publicfiles/business/htmlfiles/mohfybjsqwss/s3581/200807/37439.htm (Last accessed 21 Aug 2017).	'Midwife' was mentioned twice.
43.	3 Nov, 2008	Regulations of the management of the safety supervision of dairy products 乳品质量安全监督管理条例(国务院第536号)	MoH	http://www.gov.cn/zwgk/2008-10/10/content_1116657.htm (Last accessed 21 Aug 2017).	This policy was a response to the scandal in China of the Sanlu milk powder incident.
44.	1 Dec, 2008	Measures for the management of neonatal screening (MoH Order No. 64) 《新生儿疾病筛查管理办法》(卫生部令第64号)	MoH	http://www.gov.cn/flfg/2009-03/05/content_1251319.htm (Last accessed 1 Apr 2017).	These measures would be effective on 1st June 2009
45.	2 Feb, 2009	A recommendation strengthen rural hospital deliveries further 《关于进一步加强农村孕产妇住院分娩工作的指导意见》[卫妇社发〔2009〕12号]	MoH	http://www.moh.gov.cn/publicfiles/business/htmlfiles/mohfybjsqwss/s3581/200902/38943.htm (Last accessed 21 Aug 2017).	Oxytocin, intravenous infusion and antibiotics were basic medications recommended to be used in normal labour and birth
46.	2 Feb, 2009	2015年80%以上农村孕产妇将住院分娩	MoH	http://www.moh.gov.cn/publicfiles/business/htmlfiles/mohfybjsqwss/s3581/200902/38942.htm (Last accessed 21 Aug 2017).	Hospital delivery rates will be above 95%, 85% & 80% by 2015 in the eastern, central & western provinces in China
47.	9 Feb, 2009	The reply of the Ministry of Health on the issue of neonatal death due to medical malpractice 卫生部关于医疗事故技术鉴定中新生儿死亡认定有关问题的批复	MoH	http://www.moh.gov.cn/publicfiles/business/htmlfiles/mohyltwjgs/s3581/200902/39050.htm (Last accessed 21 Aug 2017).	See: 'Regulations of Medical Malpractice' (2002-4-4)

(Continued)

Table 3.2 (Continued)

	Date	Policy	Department	Sources	Interpretation
48.	24 Jun, 2009	The protocol of giving folic acid to prevent neural tube defects 增补叶酸预防神经管缺陷项目管理方案	MoH	http://www.moh.gov.cn/publicfiles/business/htmlfiles/mohfybjysqwss/s3581/200906/41532.htm (Accessed 21 Aug 2017).	Rural women could get free folic acid since 2009
49.	16 Sep, 2009	The assessment of neonatal deaths (Trial) [2009] No. 109 《新生儿死亡评审规范（试行）》卫妇社儿卫便函（2009）109号	MoH	http://www.moh.gov.cn/publicfiles/business/htmlfiles/mohfybjysqwss/s3585/200910/43159.htm (Last accessed 21 Aug 2017).	'Midwife' is mentioned twice and is identified with nurses and birth attendants. Two survey forms are attached
50.	16 Nov, 2009	National work plan for neonatal screening, (No 64) 《全国新生儿疾病筛查工作规划》（卫生部第64号部长令)	MoH	http://www.moh.gov.cn/publicfiles/business/htmlfiles/mohfybjysqwss/s3585/200911/44716.htm (Last accessed 21 Aug 2017).	Regular neonatal screening should be conducted in accordance with the MoH.
51.	1 Dec, 2010	The neonatal screening technical specifications (2010 Edition) 新生儿疾病筛查技术规范（2010版）	MoH	www.moh.gov.cn/cmsresources/mohfybjysqwss/.../doc10798.doc (Last accessed 21 Aug 2017).	Increase assessment and evaluation
52.	10 Jan, 2011	The pathway of placenta previa and other six obstetric complications issued by the General Office of the Ministry of Health. 卫生部办公厅关于印发完全性前置胎盘等产科7个临床路径的通知	MoH	http://www.moh.gov.cn/publicfiles/business/htmlfiles/mohyzs/s3586/201101/50314.htm (Last accessed 21 Aug 2017).	Attempted to standardize the protocol for these seven obstetric complications.
53.	11 Apr, 2011	'The standards and requirements of the quality of maternal health services in urban and rural areas' & other six rules were revoked by the Ministry of Health (Decree Order 83).	MoH	http://www.moh.gov.cn/mohzcfgs/s3576/201107/52263.shtml (Last accessed 31 Mar 2017).	Documents revoked 1985.6.1 1985.6.30 1986.6.30 1987.4.7 1989.2.10 1989.20.10 1996.8.27

No.	Date	Title	Source	URL	Notes
		卫生部决定废止《全国城乡孕产期保健质量标准和要求》等7件部门规章			No relevant replacement regulations/laws have been enacted since then. This poses a great danger for the public, esp. Home births
54.	23 Jun, 2011	'The management of maternal health care' and 'the standards of maternal health care,' 《孕产期保健工作管理办法》和《孕产期保健工作规范》卫妇社发（2011）56号	MoH	http://www.nhfpc.gov.cn/zwgkzt/glgf/201306/61f0bee3af344623a566ab099ffbf34.shtml (Last accessed 1 Apr 2017).	Maternity care period defined as from conception to 42 days postnatally. No mention of midwife but birth attendants
55.	8 Aug, 2011	Development of Chinese Women and Chinese children (2011-2020) 中国妇女发展纲要和中国儿童发展纲要(2011-2020)[国发（2011）]	MoH	http://www.gov.cn/gongbao/content/2011/content_1927200.htm (Last accessed 21 Aug 2017).	The development will be assessed annually and and at the beginning and end of the project.
56.	31 Dec, 2011	Nursing career development program (2011-2015) 中国护理事业发展规划纲（2011-2015年）	MoH	http://www.moh.gov.cn/mohyzs/s3593/201201/53897.shtml http://www.gov.cn/gzdt/2012-01/10/content_2040677.htm (Last accessed 21 Aug 2017).	The target number of registered nurses by 2015 will be 2,860,000
57.	8 Feb, 2012	Maternal and child health literacy - the basic knowledge and skills (Trial) 《母婴健康素养：基本知识与技能(试行)》	MoH	http://www.moh.gov.cn/publicfiles/business/htmlfiles/mohfybjysqwss/s3589/201202/54080.htm (Last accessed 21 Aug 2017).	Balanced diet is important for health.
58.	17 Feb, 2012	The notice of the The The implementation and development notice of China's women and children program 2011-2020. [MoH 2012] No. 12 2011-2020年中国妇女儿童发展纲要实施方案的通知(卫妇社发（2012）12号)	MoH	http://www.nhfpc.gov.cn/fys/s7900/201202/cffcb29c192d4e529c6290c280507df9.shtml (Last accessed 1 Apr 2017).	It is an important part of the study. Main targets: Maternal mortality rate 2015: 22/100,000, 2020: 20/100,000. Fetal mortality rate: 2015: 12-14/1000, 2020: 10-13/1000. Urban hospital births >98%, Rural hospital births>96% No mentioning midwife

(Continued)

Table 3.2 (Continued)

	Date	Policy	Department	Sources	Interpretation
59.	28 Apr, 2012	The guidance of the Ministry of Health on the implementation of the management of hospital nurse jobs 卫生部关于实施医院护士岗位管理的指导意见 卫医政发（2012）30号	MoH	http://www.moh.gov.cn/mohyzs/s3593/201205/54600.shtml (Last accessed 21 Aug 2017).	The ratio of care bed & nurse is not less than 0.4:1, ICU nurse-patient ratio as 2.5-3:1 the neonatal intensive care unit nurse-patient ratio 1.5-1.8:1
60.	2 May, 2012	Standards for the health visits of the newborns 新生儿访视等儿童保健技术规范	MoH	http://www.moh.gov.cn/publicfiles/business/htmlfiles/mohfybjysqwss/s3585/201205/54596.htm (Last accessed 21 Aug 2017).	There are four relevant documents but unfortunately they are inaccessible.
61.	17 Feb, 2012	The implementation and development of the 2011-2020 outline for China's women and children of the Ministry of Health 卫生部关于印发贯彻2011-2020年中国妇女儿童发展纲要实施方案的通知.卫妇社发（2012）12号	MoH	http://www.moh.gov.cn/mohfybjysqwss/s7900/201202/54194.shtml (Last accessed 21 Aug 2017).	'Midwife' was mentioned twice. There are five sections. MMR is to be reduced to 15% compared with the previous year and the infant mortality, down 10 %
62.	10 Apr 2017	Evaluation criteria for Levels 3 maternal and child health hospitals 三级妇幼保健院评审标准（2016年版）	National Health & Family Planning Commission (NHFPC)	http://www.nhfpc.gov.cn/fys/s3581/201609/1dce4771f1664571 8e0fa8741d07c98b.shtml (Last accessed 10 Apr 2017).	Refers to the hospitals at and above city, county & provincial levels. 'Midwife' was mentioned twice.
63.	10 Apr 2017	Evaluation criteria for Levels 2 maternal and child health hospitals 二级妇幼保健院评审标准（2016年版）	NHFPC	http://www.nhfpc.gov.cn/fys/s3581/201609/1dce4771f1664571 8e0fa8741d07c98b.shtml (Last accessed 10 Apr 2017).	Refers to the hospitals below city, county & provincial levels. 'Midwife' was mentioned twice.

The International Confederation of Midwives Gap Analysis Workshop in China

Background

The iatrogenic nature of maternity care in China, apparent in the poor maternal, fetal and neonatal outcomes, is associated with the medicalisation of the services, a change which is linked to the marginalisation and demise of midwifery. This problem was addressed in a workshop organised by the Midwifery Research Unit in *Hángzhōu* Normal University, China, and the International Confederation of Midwives (ICM), together with other stakeholders. The Workshop focused particularly on education, regulation and the development of a professional association for midwives. The objectives were to identify gaps in these three areas with a view to re-establishing midwifery in China. Sixty participants representing a range of governmental, professional and non-governmental organisations were invited. The significance of this innovative event, for Chinese midwifery and for midwifery globally, cannot be overstated. ICM tools were employed and improved using research findings, where available.

Gaps identified by the assessment of the ICM Gap Analysis Workshop

Key: 0 Not present, needs to be developed
- • Needs much strengthening
- ▲ Needs some strengthening
- ◎ Already present/no action needed

Education	Situation analysis (Strengths, weakness/ gaps)	Priority Actions
• National education policy 0 Definition of midwife 0 Registered midwife 0 Community midwife 0 Community extension worker 0 Standards-based curriculum 0 University degree courses 0 Workforce statistic • Teacher training ◎ Secondary midwifery education	✧ Midwifery education is subsumed under nursing. ✧ Secondary vocational school education only ✧ No national policy or mechanism to regulate despite regular and well-functioning facility reporting system. ✧ Absences of a vision, a mission, national policies, standards and deployment systems for midwives after graduation from midwifery education programme	✧ Study the ICM and World Health Organization definition of a midwife ✧ Develop standards of education ✧ Develop midwifery BSc, MSc and PhD education ✧ Develop standards ✧ Improve curriculum ✧ Adjust the right ratio of theoretical studies & clinical practice in education system. ✧ Control quality of teaching and reflexive and transformational learning

(Continued)

(Continued)

Education	Situation analysis (Strengths, weakness/ gaps)	Priority Actions
Regulation	Situation analysis (Strengths, weakness/ gaps)	Priority Actions
0 ICM definition of midwife 0 Registered & enrolled midwife 0 Community midwife 0 National plan 0 Legislation/ regulation mechanism 0 National specific policy for midwifery and midwives 0 Notification to practice 0 A register of midwives 0 Capacity to review and act 0 Midwifery professional/career ladder ◎ Secondary midwifery education ▲ Review of the system ▲ Midwife-led care	✧ China does not use ICM definition ✧ Acute shortage of midwives ✧ No legislation that recognises midwifery as an autonomous regulated profession ✧ Legislation does not have a transparent process for nomination, selection and appointment to the regulatory authority and identifies roles and terms of appointment. ✧ Not all key stakeholders involved in the operational planning process ✧ The first midwife-led normal birth unit promotes vaginal births with caesarean section rates <10% & it leads to an ongoing randomised controlled trials study in 10 hospitals but needs national policy commitments	Develop ✧ national legislation ✧ national policies on midwifery ✧ a register for midwives and open it to the public ✧ a mechanism for a range of registration ✧ a professional career ladder ✧ standards for education ✧ standards for regulation ✧ standards for association ✧ standards for midwifery practices ✧ a review system ✧ an audit system ✧ a code of conduct ✧ capacity-building mechanism
Association	Situation analysis (Strengths, weakness/gaps)	Priority Actions
0 national midwives association • 2 provincial midwives associations • Midwifery Expert Committee (MEC), Chinese Maternal and Child Health Association (CMaCHA)	✧ The number and activities of each provincial association, MEC and CMCHA are unclear.	✧ Study MACAT ✧ Discuss the necessity & possibility of establish a national association ✧ Develop constitution for a national association

Call to action

Shijiazhuang China – the International Confederation of Midwives
Midwifery Development Workshop

27th March 2014
We, the participants of the Midwifery Development in China Midwifery: Gap Analysis Workshop declare our commitment to the provision of high quality midwifery services which are available, affordable, accessible and acceptable to women. Our vision of this workshop is that midwives will be the lead professionals, coordinating care within a multidisciplinary team which include obstetricians, paediatricians, general practitioners, public health workers and nurses. Midwives are the backbone to maternal newborn and child health. To improve the maternity care and optimize the health outcomes of women, children and families, we call upon the government, relevant health and educational departments, policy makers, public and private sectors partners to:

- **Invest** in the strengthening of midwifery profession, in midwives education, regulation, professional association development including supporting research activities for the universal access to high quality of midwifery care. Invest in competency-based, innovative educational programmes and infrastructure that result in fully qualified and competent midwives who will promote the health of mothers, babies and families. Our attention and resources will be focused on people, not their illness, on health normal birth and delivery, not disease.
- **Educate** midwives to be woman-centred to achieve high quality of care that optimizes the health of women, newborns and their families in a changing environment. Develop midwifery education programmes which meet local needs and the Global Standards for midwifery education. Give midwives appropriate support in updating midwives' competence with on-going educational programmes and professional development. Educate the public to understand the concept of midwifery, midwives, normal labour and birth.
- **Regulate** midwifery education and licence midwives so that they are authorized and supported to provide the services they are educated for and competent to deliver within the permitted scope for women, children and families. Focus on processes for establishing a council for the development of legislation, and regulations specifically for defining the scope of practice and ethics for midwives and for the protection of the women, children, and family interests; incorporating the processes into strategic plans for national health reform. Set up policies for monitoring and evaluation to ensure the accountability of all actors for results.
- **Support midwives' associations at regional, national and international levels** to provide leadership and professional support to midwives. Support the association to contribute to the formulation and implementation of guidelines, policies and protocols for practice to enhance the ability of midwives

to meet the expectations of women and improve the health of women; set up a task force to advocate for better recognition, support, security, and working conditions including remuneration and to represent the interests of the profession.

Declared on this 27th day of March 2014 in Shijiazhuang, Hebei, China, at the Shijiazhuang China – ICM Midwifery Development Workshop.

Partner Organisations (priority and alphabetic order)

Hebei Provincial Health & Family Planning Commission
Hebei Chinese Society of Perinatal Medicine
International Confederation of Midwives (ICM)
Shijiazhuang City Health and Family Planning Commission
Shijiazhuang Maternal and Children's Hospital
Shijiazhuang City Health and Family Planning Commission
United Nations Population Fund (UNFPA)
Chengde City Maternal and Children Hospital
Chinese Physician Association
Chinese Maternal & Child Health Association
Chinese Medical Association
Chinese Society of Perinatal Medicine
Chinese Nursing Association
Fujian Provincial Maternity and Children Hospital
Guangdong Chinese Society of Perinatal Medicine
Guangdong Maternal and Children's Hospital
Guangdong Provincial Midwifery Association
Hángzhōu Maternal and Children Hospital, *Zhèjiāng* Province
Hainan Medical College
Handan City Maternity and Children Hospital
Handan Central Hospital
Hebei Armed Police Corps Hospital
Hengshui City Maternal and Children Hospital
Jinhua Professional Technology Medical College
Jinbao Women & Children Hospital
Liuan City of Anhui Province Hospital, Anhui Province
Luanping County Maternity and Children Hospital
Luzhou People's Hospital, Sichuan Province
Midwifery Expert Committee, Chinese Maternal & Child Health Association
National Centre of Maternal and Children Health
National Health and Family Planning Commission of the People's Republic of China
Ningjin Country Western and Chinese Medicine Combined Hospital
No. 302 Army Hospital
Peking Union Medical College Hospital

Putian Nursing College, Fujian Province
Qinhuangdao Maternity and Children Hospital
Raoyang County Hospital, Hebei Province
Shenzhen Baoan Maternal and Children Hospital
School of Nursing, *Hángzhōu* Normal University
Tianjin Medical University
Yongnian County Maternity and Children Hospital
Zhèjiāng Midwives Association

References

AAT (Association of Accounting Technicians). 2014. AAT code of professional ethics. www.aat.org.uk/sites/default/files/assets/AAT_Code_of_Professional_Ethics.pdf (Last accessed 12 July 2015).

Ahern, E.M. 1978a. Chinese-style and western-style doctors in Northern Taiwan. In: Kleinman, A., Kunstadter, P., and Alexander, E.R et al. (eds.) *Culture and Healing in Asian Societies*. Schenkman Publishing Company, Cambridge, MA: 101–111.

Ahern, E.M. 1978b. Sacred and secular medicine in a Taiwan village: A study of cosmological disorder. In: Kleinman, A., Kunstadter, P., and Alexander, E.R. et al. (eds.) *Culture and Healing in Asian Societies*. Schenkman Publishing Company, Cambridge, MA: 17–40.

Ahern, E.M. 1978c. The power and pollution of Chinese women. In: Wolf, A.P. (ed.) *Studies in Chinese Societies*. Stanford University Press, Stanford: 269–290.

Anderson, E.N. 1988. *The Food of China*. Yale University Press, New Haven.

Andrews, B., and Bullock, M.B. (eds.). 2014. *Medical Transitions in Twentieth Century China*. China Medical Board Centennial Series. Indiana University Press, Indiana. https://muse.jhu.edu/chapter/1339077 (Last accessed 17 March 2017).

Annandale, E. 2009. *Women's Health and Social Change*. Routledge, London.

Antonovsky, A. 1979. *Health, Stress, and Coping*. Jossey-Bass Publishers, San Francisco.

Antonovsky, A. 1987. *Unraveling the Mystery of Health – How People Manage Stress and Stay Well*. Jossey-Bass Publisher, San Francisco.

Arms, S. 1994. *Immaculate Deception II – Myth, Magic and Birth*. Celestial Arts, Berkeley, CA.

Barnard, A. 2000. *History and Theory in Anthropology*. Cambridge University Press, Cambridge.

Barnard, A., and Spencer, J. (eds.). 2002. *Encyclopaedia of Social and Cultural Anthropology*. Routledge, London.

Beech, B.A.L. 2008. Making normal birth a reality. *AIMS Journal* 20(4): 9. www.aims.org.uk/Journal/Vol20No4/makingNormalBirthAReality.htm (Last accessed 02 May 2017).

Beech, B.A.L., and Phipps, B. 2008. Normal birth: Women's stories. In: Downe, S. (ed.) *Normal Childbirth: Evidence and Debate* (2nd ed). Churchill Livingstone, Edinburgh: 67–79.

Běijīng Health Authority (北京市卫生局) 2004. The methods for the management of midwifery and obstetric technology in Běijīng 北京市助产技术管理办法. www.doc88.com/p-5807176094205.html (Last accessed 14 March 2017).

Berger, P.L. 1966. *Invitation to Sociology*. Penguin, Harmondsworth.

BHMCHH (Beijing Haidian Maternal and Child Health Hospital 北京海淀区妇幼保健院). 2015. Family planning technical guidance centre 计划生育技术指导中心. www.

guahao.com/hospital/introduction/FF0153A8F0272010E0430F01A8C07495000 (Last accessed 02 May 2017).

Black, J. (ed.). 1999. *DK Atlas of World History: Mapping the Human Journey.* Dorling Kindersley Limited, London.

BMCH (Baijia Maternity Care Holdings). 2014. *Baijia on the Way.* Baijia Maternity Care Holdings, China.

Braverman, H. 1975. *Labour and Monopoly Capital: The Degradation of Work in the Twentieth Century.* Monthly Review Press, New York.

Bruce, S. 2000. *Fundamentalism.* Polity Press, Cambridge.

Bruyn, S.T. 1966. *The Human Perspective in Sociology: The Methodology of Participant Observation Englewood Cliffs.* Prentice-Hall Inc, Englewood Cliffs, NJ.

Burgess, R.G. (ed.). 1982. *Field Research: A Source Book and Field Manual: Issue 4 of Contemporary Social Research Series.* Routledge, London.

Bynum, W., and Bynum, H. 2011. *Great Discoveries in Medicine.* Thames & Hudson, London.

Byrom, S., Byrom, A., and Downe, S. 2011. Transformational leadership and midwifery: A nested narrative review. In: Downe, S., Byrom, S., and Simpson, L. (eds.) *Essential Midwifery Practice- Leadership, Expertise and Collaborative Working.* Wiley-Blackwell, Oxford: 23–43.

Cai, H. (蔡鸿源) (ed.). 1999. *Collection of Legislation of the Republic of China.*《民国法规集成》Vol 26 Huangshan Publishing Society. Hefei (合肥黄山书社).

Cai, M.M., Marks, J.S., Chen, C.H., Zhuang, Y.X., Morris, L., and Harris, J.R. 1998. Increased cesarean section rates and emerging patterns of health insurance in Shanghai, China. *American Journal of Public Health* 88(5): 770–80.

Campbell, R. 1997. Place of birth reconsidered. In: Alexander, J., Levy, V., and Roth, C. (eds.) *Midwifery Practice: Core Topics*, vol.2. Macmillan Press, Suffolk.

Campbell, R., and Macfarlane, A.J. 1996. *Evaluation of the Midwife-Led Maternity Unit at the Royal Bournemouth Hospital: Final Report to the Dorset Health Commission.* NPE, Oxford.

Carr, E.H. 1986. *What Is History?* (Reprinted 2001) Palgrave Macmillan, Houndmills, Basingstoke.

Carr-Saunders, A.M., and Wilson, A.P. 1933. *The Professions.* Clarendon Press, Oxford.

CCTV (中央电视台) 2005. The revolution of birth. (生育革命) *CCTV.* www.cctv.com/life/38/20fzs05.html (Last accessed 02 June 2006).

CEEC (Chinese Encyclopaedia Editing Committee). 1979. Chinese Encyclopaedia《百科知识全书》.CEEC (中国大百科全书总编辑委员会), *Shànghǎi* Dictionary Publishing House, Shànghǎi.

Chang, C.C. (常存库) 2003. *Chinese Medical History.*《中国医学史》Chinese Medicine and Pharmacology Press，Běijīng.

Chang, X., and Lu, H. 2013. Investigation and study on current situation and influencing factors for core midwifery competency in Beijing. *Maternal & Child Health Care of China*中华妇幼保健 38(9): 1462–5. www.doc88.com/p-0806893604568.html (Last accessed 29 June 2017).

Chén, Z.M. (陈自明) 1237 *Fùrén dàquán Liáng fāng* 《妇人大全良方》24 Vols, (The Complete Effective Prescriptions for Married Women) In: *Sì-kù-quán-shū*: Medicine 48: 742 (*Sì-kù* Complete Collection: Medicine 48: 742) (Reprinted 1987).《四库全书：子部，医家类48》*Shànghǎi* Ancient Books Publishing House, *Shànghǎi* 742: 435–800.

Cheung, N.F. 1996a. Background and cosmology of Chinese diet therapy in childbearing. *Midwives* 109(1301): 190–193.

Cheung, N.F. 1996b. Postnatal diet therapy from a Chinese perspective. *Midwives* 110(1302):146–149.

Cheung, N.F. 1997. Chinese *Zuo yuezi* in Scotland. *Midwifery* 13(2): 55–65.

Cheung, N.F. 2009. Chinese midwifery: The history and modernity. *Midwifery* 25(3): 228–241.

Cheung, N.F. 2015. Making it happen in China. In: Byrom, S. and Downe, S. (eds.) *The Roar Behind the Silence*. Pinter & Martin Publishers. www.pinterandmartin. com/blog/the-roar-behind-the-silence-published-october-2014/ (Last accessed 16 February 2015).

Cheung, N.F., and Fleming, A. 2011. Case studies of collaboration in the UK and China. In: Downe, S., Byrom, S., and Simpson, L. (eds.) *Essential Midwifery Practice – Leadership, Expertise and Collaborative Working*. Wiley-Blackwell, Oxford: 180–194.

Cheung, N.F., Mander, R., and Cheng, L. 2005a. The 'doula-midwives'. *Shànghǎi Evidence Based Midwifery* 3(2): 73–79.

Cheung, N.F., Mander, R., Cheng, L., Chen, V.Y., Yang, X.Q., Qian, H.P., Qian, J.Y. 2006. 'Zuoyuezi' after caesarean in China: an interview survey. *International Journal of Nursing Studies* 43(2): 193–202.

Cheung, N.F., Mander, R., Cheng, L., Yang, X.Q., and Chen, V.Y. 2005b. 'Informed choice' in the context of caesarean decision-making in China. *Evidence Based Midwifery* 3(1): 33–38.

Cheung, N.F., Mander, R., Cheng, L., Yang, X.Q., and Chen, V.Y. 2006. Caesarean decision-making: Negotiation between Chinese women and healthcare professionals. *Evidence Based Midwifery* 4(1): 24–30.

Cheung, N.F., Mander, R., *Wáng*, X., Fu, W., and Zhu, J. 2009a. Chinese midwives' views on a midwife-led normal birth unit. *Midwifery* 25(6): 744–755. www.midwiferyjournal. com/article/S0266-6138(10)00144-0/abstract (Last accessed 23 January 2011).

Cheung, N.F., Mander, R., *Wáng*, X., Fu, W., and Zhu, J. 2009b. The planning and preparation for a 'homely birthplace' in *Hángzhōu*, China. *Evidence Based Midwifery* 7(3): 101–106.

Cheung, N.F., Mander, R., *Wáng*, X., Fu, W., and Zhu, J. 2011a. Views of Chinese women and health professionals about the midwife-led care in China. *Midwifery* 27(6): 842–847, doi:10.1016/j.midw.2010.09.001

Cheung, N.F., Mander, R., *Wáng*, X., Fu, W., and Zhu, J. 2011b. Clinical outcomes of the first midwife-led normal birth unit in China: A retrospective cohort study. *Midwifery* 27(5): 582–7. Epub 2011. January 13, 2011. http://dx.doi.org/10.1016/j.midw.2010.05.012 (Last accessed 18 January 2011).

Cheung, N.F., Chang, L.P., Mander, R., Xu, X., and Wang, X. 2011c. Proposed professional education programme for midwives in China: New mothers' and midwives' views. *Nurse Education Today* 31(5): 434–8.

Cheung, N.F., and Pan, A. 2012. Childbirth experience of migrants in China: A systematic literature review. *Nursing & Health Sciences* 14(4): 362–371. doi:10.1111/j.1442–2018.2012.00728.x. http://onlinelibrary.wiley.com/doi/10.1111/ j.1442-2018.2012.00728.x/abstract (Last accessed 14 September 2012).

China News Network (中国新闻网) 2011. The infant mortality rate of China dropped to 13/1000, achieving the UN Millennium development goals "中国婴儿死亡率降至 13/1000，实现联合国千年发展目标". http://health.people.com.cn/GB/14727448. html (Last accessed 08 November 2011).

Chinese Ministry of Education (中央教育部) 1937. Recent news on occupation 最近职业 消息 *Journal of Village Education* 乡村教育 3(184): 341–342.

Chinese Ministry of Health and Education (中央卫生部及教育部) 1951. The draft programme for Nursing and midwifery education system and courses *Zhèjiāng* Archives 关于发展卫生教育和培养各级卫生工作人员的决定 浙江省档案局 J165–1–115: 26.

Chinese Ministry of Health and Ministry of Politics (中央卫生部及政治部) 1979. Recommendations on health technology promotion关于卫生技术推广的建议. http://192.168.209.242/elaw/ApiSearch.dll?ShowRecordText?Db=chl&Id=12&Gid=33118&ShowLink=false&PreSelectId=188356080&Page=0&PageSize=20#m_font_0 (Last accessed 24 March 2008).

Chinese Nationalist Government (民国政府) 1943. Midwifery law. *Zhèjiāng* Archives: 助产士法 浙江省档案局 L029–004–0232 www.9939.com/pub/200710/11932045171.htm (Last accessed 02 June 2009) www.med66.com/html/ziliao/07/89/e9ac1f73be8c016431593514e9d70ea1.htm. (Last accessed 07 April 2009).

Chiou, Y.L., and Chou, F.H. (邱宜令, 周汎澔) 2006. The past and future of the midwifery profession and education in Taiwan 谈台湾助产专业及教育之沿革与未来展望 *Devoting to Nursing* 志为护理 5(2): 65–70.

CMoH (中央卫生部) 1928. Midwives rules《助产士条例》 Chinese Ministry of Health of the Nationalist Government. http://book.xuexi365.com/ebook/detail.jhtml?id=10817564&page=79 (Last accessed 02 December 2013).

CMoH (中央人民政府卫生部) 1952. Temporary codes and conducts for doctors, pharmacists, midwives, nurses and dentists. 医士、药剂士、助产士、护士、牙科技士暂行条例. www.jkcsw.com/hlzt/hlgl/200601/15266.html. (Last accessed 10 March 2008.

CMoH. 1999. The comparative statistics of the health workers of 1997 and 1998 in China. 1998 年全国卫生人员数与1997年比较. www.moh.gov.cn/open/statistics/jb98/t2.html (Last accessed 17 March 2017).

CMoH. 2001. The bulletin of 2001 national health statistics. www.moh.gov.cn/publicfiles/business/htmlfiles/zwgkzt/pgb/200805/34844.htm (Last accessed 02 August 2012).

CMoH. 2006a. The methods of hospital classification and its management. www.100md.com/html/DirDu/2006/08/29/15/65/16.htm (Last accessed 4 May 2007).

CMoH. 2006b. A conference paper for Women's and Children's Health in China: *Zhèjiāng* Health Authority speeded up building a healthy province and took steps to promote the development of Women and Children's Health. The Ministry of Health, the People's Republic of China. www.moh.gov.cn/newshtml/16674.htm (Last accessed 2 July 2008).

CMoH. 2008a. A questionnaire survey of midwifery resources in China 中国助产技术人力资源现况调查. www.nmwst.gov.cn/uploads/soft/6_081014082803.pdf (Last accessed 18 March 2009).

CMoH. 2008b. Mortality rate of children under 5-year in surveillance region 2008监测地区5岁以下儿童死亡率. www.moh.gov.cn/publicfiles/business/htmlfiles/zwgkzt/ptjty/digest2008/q43.htm (Last accessed 07 April 2010).

CMoH. 2009. Guide for further strengthening hospital delivery in rural areas. Ministry of Health, PR China 20th January. www.gdwst.gov.cn/a/200718wj/200908057015.html (Last accessed 01 January 2013).

CMoH. 2011a. Ministry of Health decided to revoke the standards and requirements of maternal health services in urban and rural areas and other seven departmental rules and regulations (Ministry of Health Decree No. 83) 卫生部决定废止《全国城乡孕产期保健质量标准和要求》等7件部门规章. www.moh.gov.cn/mohzcfgs/s3576/201107/52263.shtml (Last accessed 31 March 2017).

CMoH. 2011b. 2010 China health statistics yearbook. Chinese Ministry of Health. www.moh.gov.cn/publicfiles/business/htmlfiles/zwgkzt/ptjnj/year2010/index2010.html (Last accessed 17 July 2012).

CMoH. 2012. 2012 Chinese health statistics. www.moh.gov.cn/publicfiles/business/htmlfiles/mohwsbwstjxxzx/s9092/201206/55044.htm (Last accessed 18 July 2012).

CMoH, UN Children's Fund, WHO UN Population Fund, UNFPA. 2006. Joint review of the maternal and child survival strategy in China. www.wpro.who.int/NR/rdonlyres/E6C29183-BC8E-4DEF-9A50-3606032E8CB4/0/MaternalandChildSurvivalStrategyinChinaENG.pdf (Last accessed 16 December 2010).

CMoH, UNICEF, and SC (The Division of Primary Health and the Maternity and Child Welfare of the Chinese Ministry of Health, UNICEF, and The Office for Women and Children under the State Council 卫生部基层卫生与妇幼保健司、联合国儿童基金会、国务院妇幼司) 2003. (eds.). The call of life: A strategic action and prospect for a safe motherhood initiative 《生命的呼唤：母亲安全项目的策略行动和展望》 by Li, C.M., Zhang, L.M., Ye, L., *Yáng*, Q., Zhang, C.Y., Wan, Y., Liu, B., Li, S.Y., Zhang, D.Y., Song, W.Z., and Chao, B. (李长明，张黎明，叶雷，杨青，张朝阳，万燕，刘冰，李世跃，张德英，宋文珍，曹彬).

CMoH, UNICEF, WHO and UNFPA. 2006. Joint review of maternal and child survival strategies in China. www.wpro.who.int/NR/rdonlyres/E6C29183-BC8E-4DEF-9A50-3606032E8CB4/0/MaternalandChildSurvivalStrategyinChinaENG.pdf (Last accessed 16 October 2010).

CMoI (Chinese Ministry of the Interior 内政部) 1928. The management rules for birth attendants 《管理接生婆规则》 Chinese Ministry of the Interior. 27–9/356. http://book.xuexi365.com/ebook/detail.jhtml?id=10817564&page=4 (Last accessed 30 March 2017).

COST 2010. ISCH COST Action IS0907: Childbirth culture, concern, and consequences: Creating a dynamic EU framework for optimal maternity care. European Cooperation in Science and Technology. www.cost.eu/COST_Actions/isch/IS0907 (Last accessed 22 March 2018).

Countrymeters. 2015. China population. http://countrymeters.info/en/China (Last accessed 01 July 2015).

Crabtree, S. 2008. Midwives constructing 'normal birth'. In: Downe, S. (ed.) *Normal Childbirth: Evidence and Debate* (2nd ed). Churchill Livingstone, Edinburgh: 97–113.

Croll, E. 1985a. *Women and Rural Development in China*. International Labour Office, Geneva.

Croll, E. 1985b. Introduction: Fertility norms and family size in China. In: Croll, E., Davin, D., and Kane, P. (eds.) *China's One-Child Family Policy*. Palgarve MacMillan, Hampshire: 1–37.

Croll, E. 1995. *Changing Identities of Chinese Women: Rhetoric, Experience and Self-Perception in Twentieth-Century China*. Hong Kong University Press, Zed Books, London.

CSC (Chinese State Council, Announced by its President Wen JB 温家宝) 2008. Nurses act state council, the central people's government of the people's Republic of China 护士条例 中华人民共和国国务院令. www.gov.cn/zwgk/2008-02/04/content_882178.htm (Last accessed 15 March 2017).

Dai, Z. (载钟英) 2004. Discussion of how to reduce maternal mortality and caesarean section rates in Shanghai 关于如何降低上海市孕产妇死亡率和剖宫产率的讨论 *Progress Obstetrics and Gynaecology* 13(5): 322–32. www.doc88.com/p-17985510453.html (Last accessed 11 November 2017).

Davis-Floyd, R.E. 1992. *Birth as an American Rite of Passage*. University of California Press, Berkeley, CA & London.

Davis-Floyd, R.E. 1994. The technocratic body: American childbirth as cultural expression. *Social Science and Medicine* 38(8): 1125–40.

Davis-Floyd, R.E., and Sargent, C.F. 1997. *Childbirth and Authoritative Knowledge, Cross-Cultural Perspectives*. University of California Press, Berkeley, CA & London.

Davis-Floyd, R.E., Barclay, L., Daviss, B. and Tritten, J. (eds.). 2009. *Birth Models That Work*. University of California Press, Berkeley & Los Angeles, CA.

DCPBGC (Department of the Capital Police of *Běiyáng* Government of China 北洋政府京师警察厅) 1913. The provisional ban of birth attendants issued by the Department of Capital Police, *Běiyáng* Government of the Republic of China《京师警察厅暂行取缔产婆规则》. In: Cai, H. (蔡鸿源) 1999 (ed.) *Collection of Legislation of the Republic of China*.《民国法规集成》 26 Huangshan Publishing Society. Hefei: 69–70. www.iolaw.org.cn/showNews.aspx?id=51601 (Last accessed 03 April 2017).

De Vries, R., Benoit, C., van Teijlingen, E.R., and Wrede, S. 2001. *Birth by Design- Pregnancy, Maternity Care, and Midwifery in North America and Europe*. Routledge, New York.

De Vries, R., Wiegers, T.A., Smulders, B., and van Teijlingen, E. 2009. The Dutch obstetrical system vanguard of the future in maternity care. In: Davis-Floyd, R.E., Barclay, L., Daviss, B., and Tritten, J. (eds.) *Birth Models That Work*. University of California Press, Berkeley & Los Angeles, CA: 31–53.

Denzin, N.K. 1970. *Sociological Methods: A Sourcebook*. Aldine Publishing, London.

DHPCMH （Department of Health Policy in Chinese Ministry of Health 卫生部卫生政策法规司) 2007. The answers to the behaviour problems of rural midwives and doctors from the Ministry of Health The Compilation of Health Laws in the People's Republic of China (2004–2005) 卫生部关于农村接生员和乡村医生执业行为相关问题的批复 中华人民共和国卫生法规汇编(2004–2005). The Press of Law *Běijīng*: 651.

Dirks, N.B.,Eley, G., and Ortner, B (eds.). 1994. *Culturer/History: A Reader in Contemporary Social Theory*. Princeton University Press, Princeton.

DoH. 1993. *A Vision for the Future*. Department of Health, The Stationery Office, London.

DONA International. 2017. What is a doula? www.dona.org/the-dona-advantage/staff-leadership/ (Last accessed 18 April 2017).

Donnison, J. 1988. *Midwives and Medical Men, a History of the Struggle for the Control of Childbirth* (2nd ed). Historical Publications, London.

Doula, U.K. 2017. About Doula UK. https://doula.org.uk/ (Last accessed 20 March 2017).

Doulas Australia. 2004. Doulas Australia. *Australian Websites*. www.pregnancy.com.au/australian_websites.htm#Doulas (Last accessed 10 May 2010).

Downe, S. (ed.). 2004a. *Normal Childbirth: Evidence and Debate*. Churchill Livingstone, Edinburgh.

Downe, S. 2004b. Aspects of a controversy: Summary and debate. In: Downe, S. (ed.) *Normal Childbirth: Evidence and Debate*. Churchill Livingstone, Edinburgh: 173–174.

Downe, S. 2007. The uniqueness of normality. *Midwives* 10(3): 132–133.

Downe, S. 2008. *Normal Childbirth Evidence and Debate* (2nd ed). Churchill Livingstone, Edinburgh.

Down, S 2009. ISCH COST Action IS0907: Child birth cultures, concerns, and consequences: Creating a dynamic EU framwork for optimal maternity care. www.cost.eu/COST_Actions/isch/IS0907 (Last accessed 18 March 2018).

Downe, S., and McCourt, C. 2004. From being to becoming: Reconstructing childbirth knowledges. In: Downe, S. (ed.). *Normal Childbirth: Evidence and Debate*. Churchill Livingstone, Edinburgh: 3–24.

Downe, S., Byrom, S., and Simpson, L. (eds.). 2011. *Essential Midwifery Practice- Leadership, Expertise and Collaborative Working*. Wiley-Blackwell, Oxford.

EBFSAMS (Editorial Board of the First State Approved Midwifery School 第一助产学校年刊编辑委员会) 1933. The preface of the establishment of *Bǎoyīng* Office for 21 years. 保婴事务所二十一年度工作弁言. *The Annual Journal of the First State Approved Midwifery School* Chinese National Library: 10–12.

ECSC (Editorial Committee, State Council 内政部年鉴编纂委员会) 1936. *State Council Yearbook IV* 内政年鉴(四). The Commercial Press, Shangai: 206–211.

Edwards, N. 2010. Why does the Albany midwifery model work? *AIMS Journal* 22(1): 5–6. No. 1. www.aims.org.uk/Journal/Vol22No1/albanyModel.htm (Last accessed 03 May 2017).

Ehrenreich, B., and English, D. 1973. *Witches, Midwives and Nurses*. Glass Mountain Pamphlets, The Feminist Press, New York.

Ehrenreich, B. 1976. *Witches, Midwives & Nurses: A History of Women Healers*. Writers and Readers Publishing Co-operative, London.

Fei, X. (费孝通) 2007. *From the Soil: The Foundations of Chinese Society* 《乡土中国》. Jiangsu Literature & Art Publishing House, Nanjing.

Feng, X.L., Guo, S., Hipgrave, D., Zhu, J., Zhang, L., Song, L., Yong, Q., Guo, Y., and Ronsmans, C. 2011. China's facility-based birth strategy and neonatal mortality: a population-based epidemiological study. *Lancet* 378: 1493–500. Published 22 October 2011. doi:10.1016/S0140–6736(11)61096–9. www.thelancet.com/pdfs/journals/lancet/PIIS0140-6736(11)61096-9.pdf (Last accessed 11 November 2017).

Feng, X.L., Xu, L., Guo, Y., and Ronsmans, C. 2012. Factors influencing rising caesarean section rates in China between 1988 and 2008. *Bulletin of the World Health Organisation* January 1, 90(1): 30–39A. Published online 2011 October 6. doi:10.2471/BLT.11.090399 PMCID: PMC3260572. www.ncbi.nlm.nih.gov/pmc/articles/PMC3260572/ (Last accessed 19 August 2012).

Firestone, S. 1971. *The Dialectic of Sex: The Case for Feminist Revolution*. Jonathan Cape, London.

Fraser, D.M., and Cooper, M.A. (eds.). 2009. *Myles Textbook for Midwives* (15th ed). Churchill Livingstone Elsevier, Edinburgh.

Freidson, E. 1970a. *Profession of Medicine*. Mean & Co, New York.

Freidson, E. 1970b. *The Profession of Medicine: A Study of the Sociology of Applied Knowledge*. Harper & Row, New York.

Freidson, E. 1986. *Professional Power: A Study of the Institutionalization of Formal Knowledge*. University of Chicago Press, Chicago.

FNU (Frontier Nursing University) 2018. The birthplace of midwifery and family nursing in America. https://frontier.edu/about-frontier/history-of-fnu/ (Last accessed 18 March 2018).

Fù, H. (傅惠) 1986. The first state midwifery school and its school headmistress: *Yáng Chong-rui* 国立第一助产学校与杨崇瑞校长 In: The selected papers in historical material. Issue 30 文史资料选编 第30辑. www.shuku.net:8080/novels/history/ytskfcnhyj/xtyj22.html (Last accessed 24 November 2004).

Fù, S. (傅山) 1425 *Fùqīngzhǔ nǚkē: Gynaecology and Obstetrics* 《傅青主女科》 Vol 1 and Vol 2 (first published in 1827) In: *Wáng*, Y.W.(王云五) (ed.). 1966 *The Basic Collection of Chinese Ancient Books Vol 085*. Taiwan Commercial Press, Taiwan.

Fù, W.K. 傅维康 1982. The development of different categories in Chinese medicine (中医分科演变琐谈) In: *Fù*, W.K., Zhang, W.F., *Wáng*, H.F., Jia, F.H., Gao, Y.Q., and Wu, H.Z. (傅维康，张慰丰，王慧芳，贾福华，高毓秋，吴鸿洲) (eds.) *The Historical Records of Chinese Medicine* 《医药史话. *Shànghǎi* Science and Technology Printing House, Shànghǎi: 42–45.

Fù, W.K., Zhang, W.F., *Wáng*, H.F., Jia, F.H., Gao, Y.Q., and Wu, H.Z. (傅维康，张慰丰，王慧芳，贾福华，高毓秋，吴鸿洲) (eds.). 1982. *The Historical Records of Chinese Medicine*《医药史话》. *Shànghǎi* Science and Technology Printing House, Shànghǎi.

Furth, C. 1987. Concepts of pregnancy, childbirth, and infancy in Ch'ing Dynasty China. *Journal of Asian Studies* 46(1): 7–35.

Furth, C. 1999. *A Flourishing Yin: Gender in China's Medical History, 960–1665*. University of California Press, Berkeley, CA.

Gao, Y.Q. (高毓秋) 1982. The earliest medical school – '*Tài-yīshǔ*- in *Táng* Dynasty (618–907) 最早的医科学校 – 唐代太医馆 In: *Fù*, W.K., Zhang, W.F., *Wáng*, H.F., Jia, F.H., Gao, Y.Q., and Wu, H.Z. (傅维康，张慰丰，王慧芳，贾福华，高毓秋，吴鸿洲) (eds.). *The Historical Records of Chinese Medicine* 《医药史话. *Shànghǎi* Science and Technology Printing House, Shànghǎi: 135–140.

Gapminder. 2010. Maternal mortality ratio 1800–2008. (Data source: IHME (from 1980) and various historical sources (1751–1979)). www.gapminder.org/data/ (Last accessed 11 November 2017).

Geelan, P.J.M., Twitchett, D.C., Bartholomew, J.C. et al. 1974. *The Times Atlas of China*. Times Books, London.

Gelbart, N. 1993a. Midwife to a nation: Mme du Coudray serves France. In: Marland, H. (ed.). *The Art of Midwifery: Early Modern Midwives in Europe*. Routledge, London: 131–151.

Grossman, A. 2008. Exploring professional values for the 21st century: Is professionalisation always to be desired? Exploring professional value for the 21st century The Royal Society for the Encouragement of Arts Manufactures & Commerce (Founded in 1754). www.rsa.org.uk/acrobat/Grossman.pdf (Last accessed 06 February 2008).

Gu, M.Y. (顾明远) 2004. *Chinese Education System: The System of Entrance Examination in History*《中国教育大系:历代教育制度考. Hubei Education Press, Hubei.

Halde, J.P.D. 1738. The art of medicine among the Chinese. In: A Description of the Empire of China (2 Vol, n.p.) II: 183–214. In: Veith, I. (ed.). 1949 *The Yellow Emperor's Classic of Internal Medicine*. University of California Press, Berkeley, CA.

Hándān City Statistics Bureau. 2016. Bulletin of 1% *Hándān* population sampling Survey in 2015. 2015年邯郸市1%人口抽样调查主要数据公报. *Hándān* City Statistics Bureau 邯郸市统计局. http://tj.hd.gov.cn/List.asp?C-1-838.html (Last accessed 21 June 2017).

Huang, R. (黄润龙) 2016. Changes and influencing factors of infant mortality rates in China in 1991–2014. 1991–2014年我国婴儿死亡率变化及其影响因素. *Population and Society* July 32(3): 67–75. www.docin.com/p-1715417538.html (Last accessed 06 December 2017).

Haralambos, M., and Holborn, M. 2008. *Sociology: Themes and Perspectives* (7th ed). Collins, London.

Harris, A., Belton, S., Barclay, L., and Fenwick, J. 2009a. Midwives in China: 'jie sheng po' to 'zhu chan shi'. *Midwifery* 25(2)：203–212.

Harris, A., Zhou, Y., Liao, H., Barclay, L., Zeng, W., and Gao, Y. 2009b. Challenges to maternal health care utilization among ethic minority women in a resource-poor region of Sichuan Province, China. *Oxford Journals Health Policy and Planning* 25(4): 311–318. http://heapol.oxfordjournals.org/content/25/4/311.full (Last accessed 04 June 2012).

Harris, F.M., van Teijlingen, E., Hundley, V., Farmer, J., Bryers, J., Caldow, J., Ireland, J., Kiger, A., and Tucker, J. 2011. The buck stops here: Midwives and maternity care in rural Scotland. *Midwifery* 27(3): 301–307.

Hays, J. 2013. Foot binding and self-combed women in China. *Facts and Details*. http://factsanddetails.com/china/cat4/sub21/item1030.html (Last accessed 01 November 2017).

HEICNG (Health Experimental Institute of the Central Nationalist Government) 1938. The draft resolution of the Health Experimental Institute of the Central Nationalist Government中央卫生实验院提案. *Chóngqìng Archives* 0053-4-3954, Article 66

Helman, C. 2000. *Culture, Health and Illness* (4th ed). Hodder Arnold, London.

Hendry, C. 2009. The New Zealand maternity system: A midwifery renaissance. In: Davis-Floyd, F.E., Barclay, L., Daviss, B., and Tritten, J. (eds.) *Birth Models That Work*. University of California Press, Berkeley, CA: 55–87.

Hodnett, E.D., Gates, S., Hofmeyr, G.J., and Sakala, C. 2004. Continuous support for women. In: *The Cochrane Library (Issue 1)*. John Wiley and Sons, Chichester.

Homer, C.S.E., Leap, N., Edwards, N., and Sandall, J. 2017. Midwifery continuity of carer in an area of high socio-economic disadvantage in London: A retrospective analysis of Albany Midwifery Practice outcomes using routine data (1997–2009). *Midwifery* 48(3): 1–10. www.midwiferyjournal.com/article/S0266-6138(17)30151-1/fulltext (Last accessed 03 May 2017).

House of Commons Health Committee. 1992. *Second Report on the Maternity Services* (Winterton report). HMSO, London.

Hu, P.A. (胡朴安) 1922a. (Reprinted in 2007) *Humanities Series- Chinese Customs, Book 1* 《人文中国系列-中国风俗》 Jiuzhou Press, Běijīng.

Hu, P.A. (胡朴安) 1922b. (Reprinted in 2007) *Humanities Series- Chinese Customs, Book 2* 《人文中国系列-中国风俗》 Jiuzhou Press, Běijīng.

Huang, X.H. (黄醒华) 2000. The present and future of caesarean section 剖宫产的现状与展望 *The Journal of the Chinese Applied Obstetrics and Gynaecology* 《中国实用妇科与产科杂志》 16(5): 259–261.

Hundley, V.A. 1995. Cost of intrapartum care in a midwife-managed delivery unit and a consultant-led care. *Midwifery* 11(3): 103–109. www.sciencedirect.com/science/article/pii/0266613895900241 (Last accessed 20 Apr 2017).

Húzhōu Women net (湖州妇女网) 2008. The statistics of the Women's Association of Húzhōu City, *Zhèjiāng* Province, China浙江省湖州市妇联的统计数据. http://sfl.huzhou.gov.cn/article.asp?id=413&classid=16 (Last accessed 05 July 2008).

ICM (International Confederation of Midwives). 2010 (amended 2013) Essential competencies for basic midwifery practice. ICM. https://internationalmidwives.org/assets/uploads/documents/CoreDocuments/ICM%20Essential%20Competencies%20for%20Basic%20Midwifery%20Practice%202010,%20revised%202013.pdf Last accessed 18 March 2018.

ICM. 2011a. ICM Global Standards for Midwifery Regulation. International Confederation of Midwives. www.internationalmidwives.org/assets/uploads/documents/Global%20Standards%20Comptencies%20Tools/English/GLOBAL%20STANDARDS%20FOR%20MIDWIFERY%20REGULATION%20ENG.pdf (Last accessed 30 July 2015).

ICM. 2011b. International code of ethics for midwives 2011. International Confederation of Midwives. www.internationalmidwives.org/assets/uploads/documents/CoreDocuments/CD2008_001%20V2014%20ENG%20International%20Code%20of%20Ethics%20for%20Midwives.pdf. (Last Accessed 15 July 2015).

ICM. 2012. ICM strategic directions 2011–2014. International Confederation of Midwives. www.internationalmidwives.org/assets/uploads/documents/Position%20Statements%20-%20English/En-ICM%20Strategic%20Directions%202011-2014-Final.pdf (Last accessed 29 April 2013).

ICM. 2014. Strengthening midwifery globally: Position statement: Professional accountability of the midwife. International Confederation of Midwives. www.internationalmidwives.org/assets/uploads/documents/Position%20Statements%20-%20English/Reviewed%20PS%20in%202014/PS2008_014%20V2014%20Professional%20Accountability%20of%20the%20Midwife%20ENG.pdf. (Last accessed 14 July 2015).

ICM. 2017. Definition of the midwife. International Confederation of Midwives. www.internationalmidwives.org/who-we-are/policy-and-practice/icm-international-definition-of-the-midwife/ (Last accessed 14 March 2017).

ICM 2018 Advocacy. ICM. http://internationalmidwives.org/what-we-do/global-reach-of-icm/advocacy.html (Last accessed 18 March 2018).

Illich, I. 1975. *Medical Nemesis: The Expropriation of Health*. Calder and Boyars, London.

Jackson, K. 2005. Right-hand woman. In: *Women's News Clippings* March 3, 2005. www.ewomensnews.org/archives/2005/03/04/right-hand-woman/#more-876. (Last accessed 03 April 2005).

James, H.L., and Willis, E. 2001. The professionalisation of midwifery through education or politics? *Australian Journal of Midwifery* 14(4): 27–30.

Jia, F.H. (贾福华) 1982. *Huángdì-nèijìng*: The Yellow Emperor's Classic of Internal Medicine 《黄帝内经》. In: *Fù*, W.K., Zhang, W.F., *Wáng*, H.F., Jia, F.H., Gao, Y.Q., and Wu, H.Z. (eds.) *The Historical Records of Chinese Medicine* 《医药史话》. *Shànghǎi* Science and Technology Printing House, Shànghǎi.

Jordan, B. 1987. High technology: The case of obstetrics. *World Health Forum* 8: 313–318. www.lifescapes.org/Writeups.htm (Last accessed 14 March 2017).

Jordan, B. 1993/1978. *Birth in Four Cultures: A Cross-Cultural Investigation of Childbirth in Yucatan, Holland, Sweden and the United States*. Waveland Press, Prospect Heights, IL.

Jordanova, L. 2006. *History in Practice* (2nd ed). Hodder Arnold, London.

Junker, B.H. 1960. *Field Work: An Introduction to the Social Sciences*. University of Chicago Press, Chicago.

Kitzinger, S. 1990. *The Crying Baby*. Penguin, Harmondsworth.

Koblinsky, M., Conroy, C., Kureshy, N., Stanton, M.E., and Jessop, S. 2000. Issues in programming for safe motherhood. http://pdf.usaid.gov/pdf_docs/PNACK513.pdf (Last accessed 14 March 2017).

Kong, B.H. (孔北华) 2005. *Obstetrics and Gynaecology*. High Education Press, Běijīng.

Lawrence, C., and Yearley, C. 2008. Regulating the midwifery profession – Protecting women or the profession? In: Peate, I. and Hamilton, C. (eds.) *Becoming a Midwife in the 21st Century*. John Wiley & Sons, Ltd, Chichester: 261–282.

Leap, N., and Hunter, B. 1993 (reprinted 2013). *The Midwife's Tale: An Oral History from Handywoman to Professional Midwife*. Pen and Sword History, Barnsley & South Yorkshire.

Lee, J. (李贞德) 1996. Childbirth in later antiquity and early medieval China 汉唐之间医书中的生产之道 Reprinted from the Bulletin of the Institute of History and Philology. *Academia Sinica* 中央研究院历史语言研究所集刊 67(3): 533–654.

Lee, J. 1999. Woman carers between *Hàn* and *Táng* Dynasties (206BC-907AD) 汉唐之间的医疗照顾者 *The History Journal of Taiwan University* 23: 123–156.

Lee, J. 2003. Gender and medicine in Tang China (618–907AD) Asia Major Third series. Institute of History and Philology. *Academia Sinica*: Taiwan 14(2): 1–32.

Lee, J. 2005. Gender and health care in Tang Dynasty 唐代的性别与医疗. In: Deng, X.N. (邓小南) *Tangsong Nuxing Yu Shehui* 唐宋女性与社会 *Běijīng Daxue Shengtang Yanjiu Congshu* 北京大学盛唐研究丛书. *Běijīng* University, Běijīng: 415–446. http://vdisk.weibo.com/s/u8SE2Ud36GysL. (Last accessed 15 March 2017).

Lee, J. (李贞德) 2008. *Women's Chinese Curing History – Gender and Health Care Between Hàn* and *Táng Dynasties in China* 《女人的中国医疗史 – 汉唐之间的健康照顾与性别》. *Sanmin* Publishing House, Taiwan.

Leung, A.K.C. 2000. Women practicing medicine in premodern China Papers in Social Sciences Taipei: Taiwan, *Sun Yat-sun* Institute for Social Sciences and Philosophy *Academia Sinica*. Reprinted from Zurndorfer, H.T. (ed.) 1999 *Chinese Women in the Imperial Past: New Perspectives*. Brill, New York: 101–134.

Lewis, P.A. 1990 Resource allocation: Whose realism? *Journal of Medical Ethics* 16: 132–3.

Li, J., and Shi, Y. 2004. The investigation and analysis of the caesarean section rates in the seven provinces in China *Conference papers for the eighth Chinese obstetrics and gynaecology symposium/ Eighth Chinese Obstetrics and Gynaecology Symposium, Nanning*, China.

Li, M. 2016. How many are there – national colleges and universities for midwifery? 全国开设助产专业院校有哪些 *Gaosan.com*. www.gaosan.com/gaokao/70274.html (Last accessed 19 October 2017).

Li S. (李时珍) 1596. Chinese Herbal Medicine (本草纲目). In: *Sì-kù-quán-shū*: (Four Library Complete Collection) Medicine 80 《四库全书：子部医家类80》, Vol.773, (Reprinted in 1987) *Shànghǎi* Ancient Books Publishing House, Shànghǎi.

Li, S., and Guō, Q. (李师圣，郭稽中) 1127 (Reprinted in 1987). The collection of *Chǎn-yù-bǎo-qìng-fāng* 《产育保庆集方》 (The Collection of Child birthing and Rearing in Sòng Dynasty (960–1279) *Sì-kù-quán-shū*: Medicine 49 《四库全书：子部医家类49》 (The Complete collection of the Four Imperial libraries: Medicine 49) (Reprinted in 1987). *Shànghǎi* Ancient Books Publishing House. *Shànghǎi* 743: 117–148.

Li, X., and Guo, Y. (eds.). 2009. *One-Hundred-Year History of the Chinese Nursing Association*. 《中华护理学会百年史话》. People's Medical Publishing House, Běijīng: 6–12.

Liang, N.G. (梁乃桂) (ed.). 1983. *Medical Practitioners and Medical Books* 《医家与医籍》. People's Medical Publishing House, Běijīng.

Liu, H.X. (刘惠喜) 2005. *Obstetrics and Gynaecology* 《妇产科学》. The Medical Press of *Běijīng* University, Běijīng.

Liu, Y.P. (刘燕萍) 2005. The beginning of the Chinese midwifery education and maternity care 中国助产教育及妇幼保健的开端. www.huliw.com/ad/lyp/33.htm. (Last accessed 29 August 2005).

Lock, M., and Nguyen, V. 2010. *An Anthropology of Biomedicine*. Wiley-Blackwell, West Sussex.

Lumbiganon, P., Laopaiboon, M., and Gulmazoglu, A.M. et al. 2010. Method of delivery and pregnancy outcomes in Asia: The WHO global survey on maternal and perinatal health 2007–2008. www.who.int/reproductivehealth/topics/best_practices/GS_in_Asia. pdf (Last accessed 14 March 2017).

Ma, Y.F., and Cheng, G.M. (马羽飞，程国明) 2006. How were our grandparents born? 我们的祖父母是怎样出生的? *Southern City Daily* 南方都市报. www.nfmedia.com/southnews/tszk/nfdsb/gzzz/fxgz/200605180623.asp (Last accessed 14 March 2017).

MacDonald, M.E., and Bourgeault, L. 2009. The Ontario midwifery model of care. In: Davis-Floyd, F.E., Barclay, L., Daviss, B., and Tritten, J. (eds.). *Birth Models That Work*. University of California Press, Berkeley, CA: 89–117.

Macionis, J.J., and Plummer, K. 1998. *Sociology: A Global Introduction*. Prentice Hall, Harlow, England.

Mander, R. 2001. *Supportive Care and Midwifery*. Blackwell Science, Oxford.

Mander, R. 2007. *Caesarean: Just Another Way of Birth?* Routledge, London.

Mander, R. 2008. Extricating midwifery from the elephant's bed. *International Journal of Nursing Studies* 45(5): 649–653.

Mander, R. 2010 The politics of maternity care and maternal health. Midwifery. Dec; 26(6): 569-72. DOI: 10.1016/j.midw.2010.09.007.

Mander, R., and Cheung, N.F. 2006. Issues arising in the planning of a cross-cultural research project in China. *Clinical Effectiveness in Nursing* 2(S2): 212–220. Women's Health and Maternity Care Special Issue. doi:10.1016/j.cein.2006.09.001 (Last accessed 27 October 2007).

Mander, R., Cheung, N.F., *Wáng*, X.L., *Fù*, W., and *Zhū*, J.H. 2009. Beginning an action research project to establish a midwife-led normal birthing unit in China. *Journal of Clinical Nursing* 19(3–4): 517–526.

Mann, M. 1983. *MacMillan Student Encyclopaedia of Sociology*. MacMillan Press, London.

Marland, H. (ed.). 1993. *The Art of Midwifery: Early Modern Midwives in Europe*. Routledge, London.

Marsh, I., Keating, M., Eyre, A., Campbell, R., and Mckenzie, J. 1996. *Making Sense of Society: An Introduction to Sociology*. Longman, London.

MCHDMH (Maternity and Child Health Department of the Ministry of Health of PRC 卫生部妇幼卫生司). 1991. Dr *Yáng Chóngruì* – The pioneer to initiate Chinese modern time maternity-child health cause 开创中国现代妇幼卫生事业的先驱杨崇瑞博士. *Journal of Maternity and Child Health* 6(6): 3–5.

MCOHK (Midwives Council of Hong Kong). 2014. Midwives registration ordinance Midwives council of Hong Kong. www.mwchk.org.hk/docs/information_to_applicants_e. pdf (Last accessed 13 March 2017).

Mei, R.L. (梅人朗) 1983. The comparision of nursing education among 25 European areas 欧洲地区25国护理教育的比较. *The Journal of International Nursing 1*国际护理学杂志：1.

MIDIRS. 1996. Support in labour. In: *Informed Choice for Professionals*. MIDIRS and the NHS Centre for Reviews and Dissemination. London.

MIDIRS. 2005. *Informed Choice for Professionals*. MIDIRS and the NHS Centre for Reviews and Dissemination. London.

MOGS (Municipality of Greater *Shànghǎi* 上海特别市政府卫生局). 1928a. (Chinese) Provisional regulations governing the registration of midwives 《上海特别市政府卫生局管理助产女士（产婆）暂时章程》 *First Register of Medical Practitioners*. Municipality of Greater *Shànghǎi, Shànghǎi* Archives: Y8–155: 179–182.

MOGS (Municipality of Greater *Shànghǎi* 上海特别市政府卫生局). 1928b. (Chinese) The first register of midwives in *Shànghǎi* by the municipality of greater *Shànghǎi* (上海特别市政府卫生局第一次登记助产女士名录) Municipality of Greater *Shànghǎi*. *Shànghǎi* Archives: Y8–155: 183–191.

MOGS (Municipality of Greater *Shànghǎi*上海特别市市政府卫生局). 1928c. (English Translation) Provisional regulations governing the registration of midwives 《上海特别市市政府卫生局管理助产女士（产婆）暂行章程》. *First Register of Medical*

Practitioners. The Public Health Bureau of the Municipality of Greater *Shànghǎi*, *Shànghǎi* Archives: U1–16–304: 1–4.

Murphy-Black, T. 1992. Systems of midwifery care in use in Scotland. *Midwifery* 8(3): 113–124.

Nánjīng Advanced State Approved Midwifery School (南京国立中央高级助产职业学校) 1936. The Midwifery Regulations of *Nánjīng* Advanced State Approved Midwifery School《国立中央高级助产职业学校章程》 *Shànghǎi* Archives: Y8–1–56–207.

NBoSoC (National Bureau of Statistics of China 中国国家统计局) 1996a. 19-11 Health care institutions. In: *China Statistical Yearbook 1996*. NBoSoC. http://www.stats.gov.cn/english/statisticaldata/yearlydata/YB1996e/S19-11e.htm. (Last accessed 20 March 2018).

NBoSoC 1996b. 19-17 Health care institutions, Beds and personnel by type of institutions 1995. In: *China Statistical Yearbook 1996*. NBoSoC. http://www.stats.gov.cn/english/statisticaldata/yearlydata/YB1996e/S19-17e.htm (Last accessed 20 March 2018).

NBoSoC 2002.1998 statistical bulletin on national and social development.《中华人民共和国1998年国民和社会发展统计公报》 http://www.stats.gov.cn/tjsj/tjgb/ndtjgb/qgndtjgb/200203/t20020331_30012.html (Last accessed 19 March 2018).

NBoSoC 2017. China statistical yearbook 2017 《中国统计年鉴》. Section 22–2 Employed persons in health care institutions. National Bureau of Statistics of China. www.stats.gov.cn/tjsj/ndsj/2017/indexeh.htm (Last accessed 11 January 2018).

NBoSoC 2003. China statistical yearbook 《中国统计年鉴》 2003, No.22. Běijīng: China Statistics Press. www.stats.gov.cn/tjsj/ndsj/yearbook2003_c.pdf. (Last accessed 05 December 2011).

Needham, J., and Lu, G. 1969. Chinese medicine. In: Poynter, F.N. (ed.) *Medicine and Culture*. Wellcome Institute of the History of Medicine, London: 255–285.

Nettleton, S. 2001, *The Sociology of Health and Illness*. Polity Press, Cambridge.

NHFPC (National Health and Family Planning Commission of the People's Republic of China). 2013. China health and family planning statistics yearbook 《中国卫生和计划生育统计年鉴》. www.nhfpc.gov.cn/htmlfiles/zwgkzt/ptjnj/year2013/index2013.html (Last accessed 05 December 2017).

NHFPC. 2016. The 2015 statistic bulletin published by the NHFPC 国家卫计委发布2015年卫生和计划生育事业发展统计公报. http://news.xinhuanet.com/health/2016-07/21/c_129166225.htm (Last accessed 06 November 2017).

NICE. 2007. Intrapartum care: Care of healthy women and their babies during childbirth. NICE clinical guideline 55 Developed by the National Collaborating Centre for Women's and Children's Health. www.nice.org.uk/CG055publicinfo (Last accessed 12 November 2007).

Nimmo, D. (ed.). 2000. Communication yearbook 3. International Communication Association. http://books.google.co.uk/books?id=rWBCpXlOLqsC&printsec=frontcover&source=gbs_navlinks_s (Last accessed 15 July 2009).

Ningxia Daily (宁夏日报) 2006. A beautiful centennial journey "世纪之旅,如此美丽" *Ningxia Daily*. www.xinhuanet.com/chinanews/2006-01/23/content_6108291.htm (Last accessed 07 July 2006).

NMC (Nursing and Midwifery Council). 2002. *Midwives Rules and Standards*. Nursing and Midwifery Council, London. www.cmft.nhs.uk/media/299676/nmc%20midwives%20rules%20and%20standards.pdf (Last accessed 17 March 2017).

Nunn, J. 2005. Canadian pulse: Doula conference. *The Canadian Women's Health Network*. www.cwhn.ca/network-reseau/2-3/pulse.html (Last accessed 02 May 2005).

O'Brien, M. 1981. *The Politics of Reproduction*. Routledge & Kegan Paul, London.

Oakley, A. 1976. Wise woman and medicine man: Changes in the management of childbirth. In: Miechell, J. and Oakley, A. (eds.) *The Right and Wrong of Women*. Penguin, Harmondsworth.

Oakley, A. 1980. *Women Confined: Towards a Sociology of Childbirth*. Martin Robertson, Oxford.

Oakley, A. 1987. From walking wombs to test-tube babies. In: Stanworth, M. (ed.) *Reproductive Technologies: Gender, Motherhood and Medicine*. Polity Press, Cambridge.

Oakley, S., and Houd, S. 1990 *Helpers in Childbirth-Midwifery Today*. Hemisphere Publishing Corporation, New York.

Ortiz, T. 1993. From hegemony to subordination: Midwives in early modern Spain. In: Marland, H. (ed.) *The Art of Midwifery: Early Modern Midwives in Europe*. Routledge, London: 95–114.

Page, L. 1988. The midwife's role in modern health care. In: Kitzinger, S. (ed.) *The Midwife Challenge*. Pandora, London: 251–260.

Pan, A., and Cheung, N.F. 2011. The challenge of promoting normality and midwifery in China. In: *Promoting Normal Birth: Research, Reflections and Guidelines*. Fresh Heart Publishing, Chester: 190–203, ISBN978-1-906619-060.

Pang, R. （庞汝彦）2010. The current situation and development of midwifery in China. 我国助产行业的现状和发展 *Chinese Journal of Nursing Education* July 7(7): 293–4.

Pang, R. 2016. China Obgy.cn's interview with Pang Ruyan in regard to the current situation and the development of midwifery in China助产专业的现状与未来. www.obgy. cn/caifangshipin/573bdcb33f4c9d2041f15d55 (Last accessed 26 October 2017).

Parahoo, K. 2006. *Nursing Research: Principles, Process and Issues* (2nd ed). Palgrave Macmillan, Houndmills, Basingstoke & Hampshire.

Parsons, T. 1951. *The Social System*. Routledge, London.

Peate, I., and Hamilton, C. (eds.). 2008. *Becoming a Midwife in the 21st Century*. John Wiley & Son, Ltd. Chichester & West Sussex.

People's Daily. 2001 Tianjin leads China's rural areas in bidding farewell to midwives. *People's Daily*. April 26, 2001. http://english.people.com.cn/english/200104/26/eng20010426_68671.html (Last accessed 09 July 2015).

People's Daily. 2002. Midwifery phase out in China's rural areas. *People's Daily*. September 30, 2002. http://en.people.cn/200209/30/eng20020930_104171.shtml (Last accessed 17 March 2017).

Petchesky, R. 1987. Foetal Image: The power of visual culture in the politics of reproduction. In: Stanworth, M. (ed.) *Reproductive Technologies: Gender, Motherhood and Medicine*. Polity Press, Cambridge.

Phillips, M.A. 2009. Women centred care? An exploration of professional care in midwifery practice. Unpublished Ph.D thesis University of Huddersfield. http://eprints.hud.ac.uk/5764/1/PhD_THESIS_MARCH_2009.pdf (Last accessed 20 April 2017).

PUMC (Peking Union Medical College 中国协和医科大学). 2018. About Peking Union Medical College. www.pumch.cn/research/gudie.html#now (Last accessed 17 March 2018).

Radcliffe, M. 1967. *Milestones in Midwifery*. John Wright and Sons Ltd, Bristol.

Renfrew, M.J., McFadden, A., Bastos, M.H., Campbell, J., Channon, A.A., Cheung, N.F., Delage, D., Downe, S.M., Kennedy, H.P., Malata, A., McCormick, F., Wick, L., and Declercq, E. (13 authors) 2014. Midwifery and quality care: Findings from a new evidence-informed framework for maternal and newborn care.*The Lancet* 384(9948): 1129–1145. www.thelancet.com/pdfs/journals/lancet/PIIS0140-6736(14)60789-3.pdf (Last accessed 16 November 2017).

Rostow, W.W. 1960. *The Stages of Economic Growth: A Non-Communist Manifesto*. Cambridge University Press, Cambridge.

Rothman, B.K. 1982. *In Labour: Women and Power in the Birthplace*. W. W. Norton, New York.

Sandall, J., Soltani, H., Gate, S., Shennan, A., and Devane, D. 2013. Midwife-led continuity models versus other models of care for childbearing women. Cochrane Pregnancy & Childbirth Group. http://onlinelibrary.wiley.com/doi/10.1002/14651858.CD004667.pub3/abstract (Last accessed 20 April 2017).

Scambler, G. (ed.). 2008. *Sociology as Applied to Medicine*. Elsevier, Edinburgh.

Schurmann, F., and Schell, O. (eds.). 1967a. *Imperial China: China Reading 1*. Penguin Books, London.

Schurmann, F., and Schell, O. (eds.). 1967b. *Republican China: China Reading 2*. Penguin Books, London.

Schurmann, F., and Schell, O. (eds.). 1967c. *Communist China: China Reading 3*. Penguin Books, London.

Seymour-Smith, C. 1986. *MacMillan Dictionary of Anthropology*. MacMillan Press, London.

Shao, L.Z. (邵力子) 1934. School journal of Shanxi provincial Midwifery School 1st Issue (陕西省立助产学校年刊首刊) *Shànghǎi*, Archives: Y8–1–1112.

Shaw, G.B. 1946. *The Doctor's Dilemma*. Penguin, New York.

Sheldon, S., and Thomson, M. (eds.). 1998. *Feminist Perspectives on Health Care Law*. Cavendish Publishing Limited, London.

Shen, M. 2008. Multi-sectorial determinants of maternal mortality in Anhui Province, China. United Nations Economic and Social Commission for Asia and Pacific. Workshop on Addressing Multi-Sectoral Determinants of Maternal Mortality in the ESCAP Region.

SHOCM (*Shèngjīng* Hospital of China Medical University 中国医科大学盛京医院). 2007. The historical review of *Shèngjīng* culture: The brief history of *Fēngtiān* Medical Unversity (*Liáonìng* Medical College) 盛京文化之历史回眸: 奉天医科大学（辽宁医学院）简史. http://baike.baidu.com/item/%E7%9B%9B%E4%BA%AC%E6%96%BD%E5%8C%BB%E9%99%A2 (Last accessed 16 March 2017).

Simpson, C.E. 1913. Does China need nurses? *The American Journal of Nursing* 14(3): 191–194. https://archive.org/stream/jstor-3404457/3404457#page/n4/mode/1up (Last accessed 11 November 2017).

Simpson, C.E. 1923 Nursing association of China. *British Journal of Nursing* September 1: 138–139 (From the Nursing Journal of India). http://rcnarchive.rcn.org.uk/data/VOLUME071-1923/page138-volume71-01stseptember1923.pdf (Last accessed 18 April 2017). http://rcnarchive.rcn.org.uk/data/VOLUME071-1923/page139-volume71-01stseptember1923.pdf (Last accessed 03 April 2016).

Smith, D.R., and Tang, S. 2004. Nursing in China: Historical development, current issues and future challenges. *Nursing in China* 5(2): 16–20. http://citeseerx.ist.psu.edu/viewdoc/summary?doi=10.1.1.470.9397 (Last accessed 16 March 2017).

Souza, J.P., Gulmezoglu, A.M., Lumbiganon, P., Laopaiboon, M., Carroli, G., Fawole, B., Ruyan, P., WHO Global Survey on Maternal and Perinatal Health Research Group. 2010. Caesarean section without medical indications is associated with an increased risk of adverse short-term maternal outcomes: The 2004–2008 WHO Global Survey on Maternal and Perinatal Health. *BMC Medicine* 8: 71. www.biomedcentral.com/1741-7015/8/71. (Last accessed 11 November 2017).

Stacey, M. 1969. *Methods of Social Research*. Pergamon, Oxford.

Stanworth, M. (ed.). 1987. *Reproductive Technologies: Gender, Motherhood and Medicine*. Polity Press, Cambridge.

Stockman, N. 2000. *Understanding Chinese Society*. Polity Press, Cambridge.

Stowell, G. (ed.). 1954. *The Book of Knowledge Volume 2 BOO-CRO*. The Waverley Book Company Ltd, London: 373–375.

Sun, M.Y. (孙美燕) 2005. *Doula Services for Childbearing Women Provided by Women's Hospital*. School of Medicine, Zhèjiāng University 浙医妇院推出导乐分娩. www.zju.edu.cn/c1429839/content_21244.html (Last accessed 02 May 2005).

Tew, M. 1990. *Safer Childbirth: A Critical History of Maternity Care*. Chapman and Hall, London.

Tew, M. 1998. *Safe Childbirth – A Critical History of Maternity Care*. Free Association Books, London.

Thurman, R. 2006. Buddha's Wheel of Life. China Image, Library of Congress. www.npr.org/programs/re/geography_heaven/kawakarpo/wheeloflife/slide.html (Last accessed 20 March 2018).

Topley, M. 1970. Chinese traditional ideas and the treatment of disease: Two examples from Hong Kong. *Man* NS Vol 5. Royal Anthropological Institute of Great Britain and Ireland.

Topley, M. 1976. Chinese traditional aetiology and methods of cure in Hong Kong. In: Leslie, C. (ed.) *Asian Medical Systems: A Comparative Study*. University of California Press, Berkeley, CA: 243–271.

Topley, M. 1978. Chinese and western medicine in Hong Kong: Some social and cultural determinants of variation, interaction and change. In: Kleinman, A., Kunstadter, P., Alexander, E.R. et al. (eds.). *Culture and Healing in Asian Societies*. Schenkman Publishing Company, Cambridge, MA: 111–37.

Towler, J., and Bramall, J. 1986. *Midwives in History and Society*. Croom Helm, London.

Tracy, S. 2007. Normal birth – What are the chances? Birth International: Specialists in Birth and Midwifery. www.acegraphics.com.au/articles/sally01.html (Last accessed 05 April 2007).

Turner, J.H. 1991. *The Structure of Sociological Theory* (5th ed). Wadsworth Publishing Company, Belmont, CA.

UNFPA, ICM, WHO et al. 2014. State of World's Midwifery 2014- A Universal Pathway. A Woman's Right to Health. UNFPA. www.unfpa.org/sites/default/files/pub-pdf/EN_SoWMy2014_complete.pdf (Last accessed 18 March 2018).

UNFPA, WHO, ICM. et al. 2011 The state of the world's midwifery – delivering health, saving lives. http://who.int/pmnch/media/membernews/2011/2011_sowmr_en.pdf (Last accessed 20 March 2017).

United Nations. 2015. Transforming our world: The 2030 agenda for sustainable development. A/RES/70/1, The United Nations. https://sustainabledevelopment.un.org/content/documents/21252030%20Agenda%20for%20Sustainable%20Development%20web.pdf (Last accessed 08 October 2016).

Unschuld, P.U. 1985. *Medicine in China: A History of Ideas*. University of California Press, Berkeley, CA.

Utumuu, L.B. 2009. Samoan midwives' stories: Joining social and professional midwives in new models of birth. In Davis-Floyd, F.E., Barclay, L., Daviss, B., and Tritten, J. (eds.) *Birth Models That Work*. University of California Press, Berkeley, CA: 119–137.

Van Gennep, A. 1909. *The Rites of Passage* (Reprinted in 1960). Routledge & Kegan Paul, London.

Veith, I. 1949. *The Yellow Emperor's Classic of Internal Medicine*. University of California Press, Berkeley, CA.

van Teijlingen, E.R. 1990. The profession of maternity home care assistant and its significance for the Dutch midwifery profession. *International Journal of Nursing* 27(4): 355–366.

van Teijlingen, E.R. 2001. Introduction to Part II. In: De Vries, R., Benoit, C., van Teijlingen, E.R., and Wrede, S. (eds.) *Birth by Design – Pregnancy, Maternity Care, and Midwifery in North America and Europe*. Routledge, New York: 115–6.

Wagner, E.D. 1994. In support of a functional definition of interaction. *The American Journal of Distance Education* 8(2): 30.

Wagner, M. 1994. *Pursuing the Birth Machine: The Search for Appropriate Birth Technology*. ACE Graphics, Camperdown, Australia.

Wajcman, J. 1991. *Feminism Confronts Technology*. Polity Press, Cambridge.

Wajcman, J. 1993. The masculine mystique. In: Probert, B. and Wilson, B.W. (eds.) *Pink Collar Blues: Work, Gender & Technology*. Melbourne University Press, Melbourne: 70.

Walsh, D. 2007a. *Evidence-Based Care for Normal Labour and Birth- A Guide for Midwives*. Routledge & Taylor & Francis Group, London.

Walsh, D. 2007b. *Improving Maternity Services: Small Is Beautiful – Lessons from a Birth Centre*. Radcliff Publishing, Oxford.

Wáng, B. (王冰注) 762 (ed.) 762 *Huángdì-nèijìng Sùwèn* (Questions on Yellow Emperor's Classic of Internal Medicine) 《黄帝内经》 (Reprinted in 1963) People's Health Publishing House, Běijīng.

Wáng, S., Wu, T., and Jin, Y. (王树楠，吴廷燮，金毓黻) 1983. *Fengtian Gazetteer: People Management and Health*. 《奉天通志_民治 卫生》 Northeast Editors Committee on Literature and History Books, 沈阳东北文史丛书编辑委员会, Shenyang.

Wáng, Z., Lin, Z., Zhao, K., Xu, Y.X., and Wu, H.M. (王忠，林战，赵坤，许玉娴，巫寒梅) 2005. The study about the relationship between midwifery care on the whole course and the quality of maternity care 全程助产责任制与产科质量关系的研究. *The Journal of Chinese Women and Children Care* 1.

Watt, J. 2004. Breaking into public service: The development of nursing in modern China, 1870–1949. *Nursing History Review* 12: 67–96.

Wei, B. (ed.). 2011. *Growing Trees Is a Ten-year Project, but Educating People Is a Lifelong Project- St. Luke's Hospital and School History*. Pútián School of Nursing, Pútián.

WHO. 1999a. *Care in Normal Birth*. World Health Organisation, Geneva.

WHO. 1999b. *Department of Reproductive Health and Research Care in Normal Birth: A Practical Guide*. World Health Organization, Geneva.

WHO. 2007. The right to health. *WHO Fact Sheet*. Joint Fact Sheet WHO/OHCHR/323. August 2007. www.who.int/mediacentre/factsheets/fs323_en.pdf (Last accessed 16 July 2015).

WHO Global Survey on Maternal and Perinatal Health Research Group. 2010. Method of delivery and pregnancy outcomes in Asia: The WHO global survey on maternal and perinatal health 2007–08. www.who.int/reproductivehealth/topics/best_practices/GS_in_Asia.pdf (Last accessed 09 December 2011).

Wintec. 2006. Unique international midwifery project. Wintec. www.scoop.co.nz/stories/GE0610/S00097.htm (Last accessed 27 April 2013).

Wolf, A.P. (ed.). 1978. *Studies in Chinese Societies*. Stanford University Press, Stanford.

World Bank, WHO, and UNFPA. 1987. *Preventing the tragedy of maternal deaths: A report on the International Safe Motherhood Conference*. World Bank, WHO, and UNFPA. Nairobi, Kenya, February 1987.

Wu, Y. 2000. The bamboo grove monastery and popular gynaecology in Qing China. *Late Imperial China* 21(1): 41–76.

Wu, X.L., and Zhang, S.M. (伍先荣, 张双梅) 1987. An investigation of the new biomedical deliveries in Badong County, Hubei Province, China 巴东县新法接生调查 *Journal of the Management of the Care of Chinese Women and Children* 2(2): 16–7.

Xia, J.S. (夏俊生) 2007. *Yáng Chóngruì* developed the maternity-child health care in China杨崇瑞开拓中国妇幼卫生事业 *The Journal of Yanhuang Spring and Autumn* 炎黄春秋 8: 36–39.

Xinhua News Agency 1980. Beijing starts up midwife classes 北京开办助产士班 *Xinhua News Agency* 新华社. 1 October 1980.

Xǔ, Y.X., and *Wáng*, Z. (许育娴, 王忠) 2005. The analysis about the relationship between midwifery care on the whole course and the quality of maternity care 全程助产责任制与产科质量的关系分析. *Chinese Primary Health Care* 1.

Yan, R. 1989. Maternal mortality in China. *World Health Forum* 10: 327–331. http://apps.who.int/iris/bitstream/10665/46871/1/WHF_1989_10(3-4)_p327-331.pdf (Last accessed 11 November 2017).

Yáng, H., and *Wáng*, H. (杨红星, 王华玲) 2007. *Yáng* Chongrui who studied abroad in the US and the modernization of Chinese health on women and babies 留美医学生杨崇瑞与中国妇婴卫生事业的近代化 *Acdemic Journal of Xuzhou Normal University* (The edition of Philosophy and Sociology) 33(2).

Yáng, J. (杨家骆) (ed.). 1967. Introduction to *Sì-kù-quán-shū* (四库全书简介). In: Li, Y.Y. and *Yáng*, J.L. (李煜瀛、杨家骆) (eds.). *Sì-kù-quán-shū Xué Diǎn* 《四库全书学典》. The Department of Chinese Dictionaries, the Institute of World Encyclopaedia, Taiwan.

Yáng, N.Q. (杨念群) 2006. *Remaking 'Patients': The Environmental Politics Under the Conflict Between Chinese Medicine and Western Medicine* (1832–1985) 《再造"患者": 中西医冲突下的空间政治(1832–1985)》. China *Renmin* University Press, Běijīng.

Yu, T. （虞抟) 1531. (reprinted in 1965). *History of Chinese Medicine* 《医学正传》. People's Health Publishing House, Běijīng.

Zhai, Y. (翟英) 2005. Doula – the friend and relative during the birth. Healthy mother 导乐 – 分娩时的朋友和亲人 健康准妈妈. http://baby.sina.com.cn/health/2005-03-03/47_69746.shtml (Last accessed 20 March 2017).

Zhèjiāng Health Authority (浙江健康委员会). 1951. The implementation plan for the training of birth attendants in *Zhèjiāng* Province 浙江省训练接生婆实施方案. *Zhèjiāng* Health Authority. *Zhèjiāng* Archives: J165–1–115: 15–16.

Zhēn, Z.Y., and *Fù*, W.K. (甄志亚, 傅维康) (eds.). 1991. *Chinese Medicine History* 《中国医学史》 *Běijīng* People Publishing House, *Běijīng*.

Zhū, D.Z. (朱端章) 1184. Practical prescriptions for the preparation of childbirth 《卫生家宝产科备要》. www.txtsk.com. (Last accessed 24 September 2010).

ZMA (*Zhèjiāng* Midwives' Association, an Affiliate of the *Zhèjiāng* Nurses' Association 隶属于浙江护理学会的浙江助产学组) 2008. *The Constitution of Zhèjiāng Midwives' Association*. ZMA, Nursing Department, Women's Hospital, School of Medicine *Zhèjiāng* University. *Hángzhōu, Zhèjiāng*, China.

Index

Note: Page numbers in *italics* indicate a figure on the corresponding page. Page numbers in **bold** indicate a table on the corresponding page.